AUTUMN'S
CHILDREN

ALAN DOELP IS THE CO-AUTHOR OF

Shocktrauma
Not Quite a Miracle

Alan Doelp

AUTUMN'S
CHILDREN

A REAL-LIFE DRAMA OF
HIGH-RISK PREGNANCY

Macmillan Publishing Company · New York

Collier Macmillan Publishers · London

Copyright © 1985 by Alan Doelp

Macmillan Publishing Company
866 Third Avenue, New York, N.Y. 10022
Collier Macmillan Canada, Inc.

Library of Congress Cataloging in Publication Data
Doelp, Alan.
    Autumn's children.
    1. Pregnancy in middle age—Case studies.
2. Pregnancy, Complications of—Case studies. I. Title.
RG556.6.D64   1985   618.3   85-2993
ISBN 0-02-532010-6

10 9 8 7 6 5 4 3 2 1

Designed by Jack Meserole

Printed in the United States of America

For Prtunick,
and Miss Alice

Contents

Acknowledgments

There is only one name on the cover of this book, but the project was a group endeavor from start to finish.

In the seminal stages of the book, Dr. Carlyle Crenshaw, Chairman of the Department of Obstetrics and Gynecology at the University of Maryland, shared his insights and chunks of his hectic schedule, and in doing so helped mold a tangle of miscellaneous information into a coherent picture of modern-day obstetrics. He also made clear his desire to share the spotlight with his two most senior colleagues, Dr. Marcos Pupkin and Dr. David Nagey, who in turn generously shared their time and knowledge.

It is only fair to point out that Dr. Crenshaw runs a sizable department, with more than a dozen full-time faculty members who teach and practice the various subspecialties of obstetrics and gynecology, but who, for reasons of time or space, appear nowhere in this book—most notably, Dr. Lindsay Alger, the fourth member of Dr. Crenshaw's team of high-risk specialists, and Dr. Maimon M. Cohen, who heads the Division of Human Genetics.

Without the cooperation of those physicians and scientists, the book could not have been written. Without the help of a great number of others, only a lesser book would have been possible. Specifically, I refer to those women who shared with me the events of their pregnancies, and with whom I now keep the compact by not mentioning their names. But they know who they are, and they will recognize pieces of themselves in the composite character of Laura Edwards.

Many others contributed valuable assistance, and I would specifically mention Trish Payne, who in a couple hours taught me as much about having babies as I'd learned from all the mothers I interviewed; Ann Jewell, who gave me an equally valuable crash course in genetic counseling; and Joanne Beisel, who guided me through the mysteries of tissue culture and karyotyping. Equally deserving of thanks are all the nurses and residents who helped; but there are too many of them to mention here, even if I could remember all the names.

Once word of the book got out, I began to receive help and advice from nearly everyone I know, and, at the risk of offending some of them, I would specifically acknowledge the contributions of Jon Franklin, Carol Benner, Dana and Dale Levitz, Kelly Gilbert, Cathy Franklin, Mark Kauffman, Maggie Kolman, and the ever-present ghost of G. Vern Blasdell.

My typing computer, a Compucorp 775, is the Rolls Royce of word processors, but even Rolls Royces require an occasional oil change. I owe special thanks to Bob Bogar, Chuck Cavolo, and Mark Zutkoff, who looked after my computer needs with unfailing efficiency and good humor.

On the business side, I owe a great deal of gratitude to Dominick Abel, who found the book a home at Macmillan, and to Arlene Friedman, whose sensitive and sensible editing brought order to a sometimes chaotic manuscript.

If success has a thousand partners, I will have no trouble sharing the credit. Whatever blame is due I will claim for my own, secure in the knowledge that the practice of having babies is likely to continue for some time, with or without my help.

ALAN DOELP

Baltimore, 1985

Foreword

This book bridges the sometimes tenuous gap between fiction and nonfiction. Its contents are the product of a year of research; the events and places it describes are real. The physicians and support personnel are likewise real, and the book uses their real names.

But the patients, all of them, are composites. Their names are invented, as are some details of their circumstances. Everything is based on the real stories of real mothers, but because of the profoundly intimate nature of the experiences they shared with me, these women did not want their names to be published, or indeed for their stories to be identifiable by friends and relatives.

So the book is, admittedly, a hybrid that will cause headaches for libraries that embrace the Dewey decimal system. I nevertheless offer it as nonfiction, because the scenery woven around the story line is all real, and because, in the course of telling this tale, I offer the reader a great deal of painstakingly documented information about the oft-misunderstood field of obstetrics.

Introduction

In a sense, obstetrics is as old as the race itself. The primates and their descendants were notable for their inclination to minister to females as they gave birth. Usually such events were painful but uncomplicated and the members of the band admired the newborn, sharing in the sense of accomplishment. Occasionally they stood and watched one of their number die in agony.

Julius Caesar was the first to decree that a dead mother's belly should be opened with a sword so that the infant inside might survive, and the operation carries his name to this day. But in Caesar's time, and for the next thousand or so years, the practice was most often futile.

Hospitals came into vogue in the centuries following the Dark Ages, but they were places that pregnant women learned to fear. Women who were delivered in hospitals, even those who had easy deliveries, often became feverish and died a few days later.

The majority of women, and certainly women of education and breeding, arranged their confinement in their own homes, attended by a midwife, perhaps, and, rarely, a doctor. The term "obstetrics" reflected medicine's love of Latin, combining the adjective *ob*, which means by or beside, with a form of the verb *stare*, which means to stand. The word captured the reality of that time, since there was little the obstetrician could do except stand by. Intervention was usually a last resort, a desperate attempt to salvage one of the two lives at stake. Occasionally, the intervention worked, and one life was saved. It was nearly always the infant's. History is riddled with the names of people who survived the birth experience but whose mothers did not.

In the eighteenth century, physicians began intervening increasingly on the mother's behalf, but often without result. Sterile technique had not yet become fashionable, and doctors spread the dreaded childbed fever from womb to womb with their unwashed hands.

Once hygiene gained acceptance, the maternal death rate dropped dramatically. But an abundance of potential complications remained. Even when the obstetrician had been relatively hygienic, often the mother developed an infection anyway and died.

Sometimes, when the mother's pelvis was too small or the child too large to pass through the birth canal, the mother would remain in labor—for days in some cases—until finally the uterus ruptured and she died quickly of hemorrhage. A few swift strokes of a knife might save the baby now and then.

If the baby was the proper size, but it came feet first and got stuck, its arms splayed out to form a sort of anchor inside the pelvis, it could usually be pulled out by the feet, but the force required sometimes broke the baby's neck. Other times it dislocated the baby's arms at the shoulders and severed a few important nerve junctions.

A baby could shift position inside the uterus, so that at term it lay with its back against the birth canal and wouldn't come out at all; and again, the mother, and usually the baby, too, would die.

Statistically, the babies survived difficult labor more often than the mothers. Mothers still bled to death following delivery, or died of a raging fever a few days later.

In the late stages of pregnancy a woman might suddenly gain weight, experience dizzy spells, blurred vision, and ringing in the ears. Later she would become remarkably nervous, a condition that lasted until delivery, or until she suddenly began convulsing. Then she usually died. It was an odd disease. Physicians thought it had something to do with the mother's blood, because of the way her blood vessels bulged toward the end, and they called it "toxemia," which means blood poisoning. It was a distressing complication, and physicians hated to see it, because they were helpless to treat it. Thankfully, it was comparatively rare.

In the early part of the nineteenth century, about 250 out of every 10,000 women died in childbirth. Bearing children was the leading cause of death in women. As medicine began to flourish in academic centers around the United States, doctors found that with aggressive treatment they could reduce the maternal death rate. Aggressive treatment meant, among other things, being willing to sacrifice the baby to save the mother's life. It is not recorded whether that judgment was first made consciously, after a sober consultation among learned specialists, or whether it simply arose from the biological reality that, in the near term, a childbearing adult is more valuable to the species than an orphaned infant.

This philosophy persisted through the nineteenth century and into the twentieth century. Its impact on the practice of obstetrics was universal and noticeable, especially in a country like the United States, which so meticulously tallies its births and deaths. By the turn of the century only about 100 of every 10,000 pregnant women died in childbirth.

Efforts were made on the baby's behalf, of course. Obstetric forceps were often useful in extricating an infant from an unyielding womb. The forceps were large, hollow, spatulate tongs that, in theory, fitted around the baby's upper head, allowing it to be pulled out by its cheekbones. Occasionally the tongs slipped, causing permanent brain damage to the baby, but on the average forceps delivery was a good thing.

Obstetricians also had to work with primitive instruments, without the benefit of blood transfusions or anesthesia. In difficult deliveries, they could sometimes reach into the womb with a cutting instrument, decapitate the fetus, and take it out in pieces. Medical instrument catalogs from the late nineteenth and early twentieth centuries offer a startling variety of instruments whose only purpose was the vivisection of unborn babies.

In the enlightenment of the twentieth century, medical and scientific knowledge blossomed and one of its earliest concerns was mortality related to childbirth. Once anesthesia had become widely available, the cesarean section was used, often successfully, even before blood transfusions were possible. A good obstetric surgeon could cut down through the abdomen, gently open the distended uterus itself, part the amniotic membrane, and lift the baby out in a gush of amniotic fluid, all in a matter of two or three frozen minutes. Happily, the amniotic fluid that flowed out into the mother's abdomen was not only sterile but even had a mysterious antiseptic property that seemed to help prevent peritonitis, which plagued patients with other types of abdominal operations. It was almost as though Nature had designed her childbearing creatures to withstand this particular surgery.

Other problems often surfaced, though, as doctors learned from their own mistakes and the mistakes of others. General anesthetics, they learned, rapidly crossed the placenta into the fetus, and the anesthetized infants often did poorly during those critical first minutes of life. Physicians learned to administer the anesthetic rapidly, the knife poised to begin the incision the instant the mother lost consciousness.

Blood loss was a problem, but rarely an insuperable one. A mother loses a full pint of blood during a normal delivery and a rapid, skillful cesarean section will cost her only two. Even before transfusion therapy became a reality, mothers bled to death less often than they once had.

The cesarean section soon proved to have a serious drawback. The long, vertical incisions, which were efficient and popular, weakened the uterine wall, and women who tried to deliver vaginally after a previous cesarean section often died in a river of blood from a burst uterus. The news spread quickly through the obstetric community, and the saying "once a section, always a section" persists today.

But, on the average, fewer women bled to death during childbirth, and the grim numbers improved even more. As maternal mortalities dropped, postpartum infection began to account for a greater and greater proportion of the death rate. The childbedfever epidemics of earlier centuries had been halted when physicians learned to wash their hands, but the problem still existed, and a significant number of women still died in the delirium of fever.

Early experience with general surgery had taught physicians that sterility was vitally important to the welfare of the patient. Applying that precept to the process of childbirth, several of the nation's most prestigious hospitals were able to report significant reductions in their postpartum infection rates. Soon, a cult of cleanliness sprang up among obstetricians. They delivered babies in operating rooms, wearing gowns and masks and sterile gloves. They carefully shaved away all traces of pubic hair from the laboring mother lest some forbidden germ be passed to mother or infant. They meticulously cleansed the mother's bowel with enemas to lessen the chance that the newborn might touch a stray piece of fecal matter. Sterile cloths were used to clean and cover the mother, antiseptics were painted all around her distended genitals, and the baby, when it emerged, was caught in a sterile towel and quickly bathed in antiseptic solutions.

It worked. By treating childbirth as a potential disaster, by taking all the same sterile precautions they took for major abdominal surgery, and by approaching the mother as a patient in need of treatment, hospitals were able to further reduce their infection rates. By the third decade of this century, only 55 out of 10,000 women died in childbirth.

Then, suddenly, came the discovery that an extract of the mold *Penicillium*, when injected into humans, could cure bacterial infections. And hematologists were reporting that transfusions of whole blood instead of plasma would soon be feasible. Every branch of medicine would benefit from the discoveries, but obstetrics seemed particularly blessed by them. In the space of two decades, the two principal complications of childbirth were wiped out. By the 1950s the maternal mortality rate had dropped to between 3 and 4 per 10,000 births, and today the rate is 0.8 per 10,000.

Obstetrics, a medical practice uniquely concerned with women, has always been shaped by society's view of those women. Reducing the maternal death rate almost to zero was a spectacular achievement. But the philosophy behind obstetrics still embodied the concept of a woman as a man's lesser partner, a man's way of reproducing himself. The death rate had begun to fall even before transfusions and antibiotics became available and much of the improvement resulted from approaching the laboring mother as though she were a valuable piece of property, like a prize mare in foal. The same women who had been taught that intercourse was to be endured as the price of having children stoically accepted the indignities and the manhandling of modern childbirth as yet another part of the sacrifice.

Even as late as the 1950s only a few women criticized the depersonalization of the birth process. The risk of infection—almost academic now, with the nearly universal use of antibiotics—loomed large in women's memories, and it seemed no more than prudent that the baby be whisked from the delivery room for antiseptic baths as quickly as the umbilical cord could be cut. Often the father saw the baby long before the mother saw either of them and for the mother it was a long, desperately lonely wait, but it would have been unthinkable for the father to enter the delivery room. Obstetricians greeted the suggestion that the father could wear a gown and mask with the kind of utter amazement a two-star general might display if he were asked to let a buck private borrow a spare uniform. And an offended doctor needed only to invoke the dread specter of infection to win any argument. Indeed, an occasional infant still developed a streptococcal infection or, worse, meningitis. The carriers of such bacteria were most likely the doctors and nurses themselves, but that reality could readily be obscured with a bit of bluster and a few big words.

The physicians who were drawn to obstetrics by the exciting discoveries of the 1930s and 1940s learned their craft in aseptic delivery suites. They received their certification and went into practice with their attitudes, skills, techniques, their very thought processes, molded forever by their teachers. There exists in medicine a profound unwillingness to tamper with anything that works and the medicine of the thirties and forties worked so well that it was still being practiced in some community hospitals in the 1960s. Even in the 1980s there are more than a few hospitals where obstetricians practice postwar medicine in postwar facilities.

But the medical schools and the teaching hospitals did not remain frozen in time. There was, as always, the quiet, scholarly, but nonetheless intense competition for achievement and peer recognition that is the driving force behind medical progress. Money is a secondary consideration; the challenge is to leave your mark on medicine. Doctors in private practice can make a very good living, if they don't mind losing sleep. But people in private practice don't win Nobel prizes; only people who do research win prizes. After the problem of maternal mortality was solved, academic obstetricians turned to fetal mortality as their new Holy Grail. And since the early 1950s, nearly all of obstetric research has centered on the developing fetus and ways to improve its odds for surviving.

At first, as in earlier times, there were comparatively few obstetricians who actively pursued research projects and those few often did so on their own time and with their own money. It was tough to argue convincingly for research funds and laboratory space when nine out of ten pregnancies needed no intervention at all and the other ten percent could usually be successfully managed in those hard, bright, surgically sterile delivery rooms.

Of course, there were birth defects and stillbirths and miscarriages, but those problems aroused little sympathy. The mothers survived, after all, and could usually try again. Medical research focused on more pressing problems, like polio, influenza, and heart disease.

Indeed, it was occasionally argued in the scientific community, why give research money for obstetrics, anyway? What good would it do? The biggest problems in obstetrics had been solved by people who had never seen the inside of a delivery room. The charge was not strictly true, but neither was it totally false. Obstetrics had always had a reputation as an intellectual backwater, a hidebound specialty concerned primarily with feeling swollen bellies, nagging the owners of those bellies about their diets, and delivering babies at all hours of the night.

As a choice of careers, obstetrics had been the traditional refuge of the lower third of the graduating class. It was routine work, work that demanded attention and even dedication, but not imagination. The prejudice against obstetrics was a medical tradition of a sort, and in those years it would not have occurred to the disparagers to wonder if part of that feeling was not a prejudice against women as well. But though it tries hard to cultivate the image, medicine is not an intellectual monolith. There are extremes of opinion in the business, and the academic catfights that go on daily are no less bitter for being couched in obfuscatory medical jargon and published in obscure medical journals. In that sense, obstetrics was no different from the rest of medicine. Its share of hidebound practitioners may have been higher than, say, neurology's, but in any major academic center there could still be found small cadres of scientists who had chosen to devote themselves to the study, and perhaps the improvement of Nature's most elegant phenomenon. The research went on in cramped quarters and with limited budgets, but it progressed nevertheless, and the results appeared in the official journals of the specialty. Bit by bit, doctors began to sort out the puzzle of what happens inside the womb.

One of the principal discoveries of the 1950s was that, if you took proper care to maintain sterility, it was possible to put a needle into the amniotic sac without damaging the fetus and draw off a small quantity of the clear yellow fluid inside. The fluid, when analyzed in a laboratory, could tell you many important things about the condition of the fetus.

Obstetric research often progressed by trial and error. The drug diethylstilbestrol, best known by its acronym DES, was used for more than twenty years to prevent early spontaneous abortions before it was suspected that DES might be linked to several rare and bizarre forms of genital cancer, not in the mother, but in the offspring. Tetracycline, one of the "miracle antibiotics," was routinely used to treat infections in pregnant women until an observant obstetrician spotted the high number of babies subsequently born with brittle bones and odd-looking gray teeth. As more and more drugs became available, obstetricians became more and more wary, and the word "teratogenic"—capable of creating birth defects—came into widespread use.

American obstetric scientists sometimes looked with envy across the Atlantic to countries like Sweden, where it was legal to terminate a pregnancy in its early stages. In the United States, before 1973, abortion was legal only in the most extreme cases—and only when the mother's life could be proved to be in danger. Abortion, even of a fetus known to be defective, was illegal. Doctors did what they could. Analysis of the metabolic byproducts in amniotic fluid provided a rich field for study and often helped physicians anticipate which babies would be born with problems that, when rapidly treated, could be manageable. The infant mortality rate showed a steady decline.

Then in 1961 President Kennedy's wife bore a premature baby that died within days. The cause of death was a condition known as hyaline membrane disease, an almost inevitable complication of premature birth. Hyaline membrane disease was neither understood nor treatable; it was simply one of the basic facts of obstetrics. Babies born too soon had underdeveloped lungs. They gasped for breath even in oxygen-rich environments, and soon died. There were theories about why, but they were only theories.

After the Kennedy infant died, the National Institutes of Health suddenly began offering very large research grants for the study of hyaline membrane disease. In the medical schools, obstetrics suddenly rippled with opportunity. It is said that the government, with its huge infusions of research grant money, exercises an influence amounting to near-total control over the direction of medical research and, while the austerity of the 1980s has made that proposition less true, it was particularly valid twenty years ago. Word spread throughout the medical schools that obstetrics was a field flush with research funds. Suddenly the cramped laboratories in the academic centers expanded into full-blown research centers and basic scientists in specialties ranging from immunology to surface physics began writing grant proposals explaining the value of their work in the field of obstetrics.

The clinicians and the research scientists approached the problem of hyaline membrane disease analytically, with clinical precision, and they found answers. In babies that were extremely premature, the tiny alveolae in their lungs were underdeveloped and collapsed each time they exhaled. Unless the next breath was a strong one, these air sacs stayed closed and no oxygen entered the baby's bloodstream.

So, doctors used respirators to feed the babies air at a slight overpressure, so that their lungs never completely deflated, and the alveolae were never allowed to collapse. Some of the babies lived. Soon hospitals all across the country built neonatal intensive-care units and, as a result, babies far sicker than the Kennedy child began to survive.

Such landmark discoveries became almost routine during the 1960s as the grant money continued to flow and obstetrics continued to attract some of the brightest scientists and clinicians to investigate the reproductive processes in ever greater detail. For the second time in thirty years, great discoveries revolutionized the field of obstetrics, but this time it was the obstetricians themselves, and not outsiders, who were doing the work.

Year by year, those physician-scientists have continued to improve the state of the art in obstetric care. Until the 1960s, babies born before the thirty-sixth week of pregnancy nearly always died. In the 1980s, it is not uncommon for babies born at twenty-six weeks to survive and develop into normal, healthy children.

With maternal deaths practically eradicated, the challenge has focused on the twin problems of infant mortality and birth defects. The definition of infant mortality is stricter in the United States than anywhere else in the world: A baby who dies after the twentieth week of gestation, or before the twenty-eighth day of life, is tallied as a "perinatal mortality." Most nations use the World Health Organization standard, in which counting does not begin until the twenty-eighth week of pregnancy and stops with the seventh day following birth. Significantly fewer deaths are tallied under those criteria, which is why, when only the officially reported mortality rates are compared, the United States appears to rank embarrassingly low among the industrialized nations of the world—somewhere around thirteenth. In fact, if the United States gathered its statistics according to WHO criteria, it would rank among the very best. But American obstetricians have set a more demanding standard for themselves. The infant mortality rate varies in different regions of the country, ranging between one and two percent. A part of that figure can be ascribed to malnutrition and neglect among pregnant women, but only a part. There are medical reasons for the rest, and obstetric scientists continue to explore ways to reduce the rate further.

The same is true of birth defects. In even the healthiest of mothers, one baby in fifty will be born with some identifiable birth defect. Pediatricians have developed ways to treat, and often cure, most of those birth defects.

Then come the high-risk factors: diabetes, high blood pressure, or heart disease in the mother; a history of genetic defects on either side of the family; late maternal age; exposure to dangerous chemicals or radiation; alcoholism, drug abuse, or malnutrition; a previous abnormal birth or births. Add those things into the equation, and the risk can go as high as one in ten.

Obstetrics, which for so long was an art, has come of age as a science. For two decades its scientists have conducted detailed studies of the factors that create high risk, and clinicians, understanding those factors, can intervene with great success. Among diabetic women, for example, the infant death rate used to be fifty percent. With modern obstetric understanding of the nature of diabetes and its effects on pregnancy, the death rate is now three percent. But even three percent, in the field of obstetrics, is high risk, and the challenge to reduce that risk continues.

The childbirth process had always been a thing of great beauty and wonder; but now that it was a respectable academic field of inquiry as well, it became commonplace to find medical students from the top third of their class choosing obstetrics as their specialty. And that new generation of medical students, the generation that came of age during the sixties, would soon begin to exert a profound influence on their chosen profession. For in the sixties it became the role, if not the obligation, of youth to point out, sometimes loudly, sometimes violently, often poignantly, the shortcomings of the body politic. And they demanded change. Civil rights should exist in reality as well as on paper. The nation should refrain from interfering in the civil wars of other nations. The community of man should take better care of its environment.

Women deserved an equal place in society.

Of all the movements that took root in the sixties, the women's rights movement was perhaps the least turbulent, but it was surely the most profound, the most far-reaching, requiring overhaul of the greatest number of society's most cherished assumptions. The same clerics who encouraged blacks to demand equality told women to love, honor, and obey their husbands. The same pacifists who picketed the White House called their girlfriends "chicks." The same biologists who described the poisoning of the biosphere pointed out that female orgasm was not essential to the reproductive process and was therefore a luxury.

Women themselves were divided on the matter. There were very few blacks who argued for a return to segregated lunch counters, but for every militant feminist there could be found an equally strident housewife. For every woman who raised the cry of job discrimination, another one argued with equal fervor that homemaking was the pinnacle of feminine achievement. For every woman who complained of sexual harassment, there was another one who pointed out that men need a lot of sex and suggested that women greet their husbands clad only in Saran Wrap.

But on the issue of childbirth, women were nearly unanimous. Something wasn't right. Something was missing. Every instinct suggested that childbirth ought to be a woman's most singular experience, and medicine had now turned it into a thing as emotionally satisfying as a tonsillectomy or an enema. At "consciousness raising" meetings the topic often occupied considerable discussion time.

One early result was childbirth classes. Women who had had babies and, still better, women who worked in delivery rooms told groups of first-time mothers what to expect. Lamaze breathing techniques, and a dozen variations, gained great popularity, and women who had given birth both with and without drugs reported that anesthesia dulled the experience as it numbed the pain. "Natural" childbirth became a slogan of women all across the country, "liberated" or not.

The obstetricians, the scientists and clinicians who had labored so furiously to apply the state of the art in science, technology, and medicine to the process of childbirth—professionals who had devoted their working lives to reducing the risk of childbearing and to improving the chances of the unborn, who indeed had invented the new specialty of high-risk obstetrics—stared open-mouthed as they were told, bluntly, that the psychology of the process was equally important, if not more so. They were shocked, at first, but they listened, and they acted.

Good scientists are flexible and imaginative; they avoid dogma and rote learning, and are always alert for new and better ways to approach a problem. The physician-scientists who, for the last twenty years, have come increasingly to dominate the field of obstetrics, are no different. Today, as the discipline of obstetrics grows ever more complex and sophisticated, the subjective experience of pregnancy and childbirth has become simpler, less overtly "high-tech," and more gratifying. The art and the science have blended together to produce a specialty that is both intelligent and caring. Medically, scientifically, and now socially as well, obstetrics has come of age.

[1]

Laurie and Bill

AFTER they made love, Laurie and Bill lay quiet for a long while. They snuggled close to each other, touching but not speaking—it was a time for reverie, not conversation. A chilly fall breeze came through the open windows, bringing with it the faintly musty smell of plants whose season is done and the monotonous drone of expressway traffic, a sound that returned magically each year when the leaves of the giant poplars grew dry and brittle and could no longer deflect it. The house stood on the north face of a gentle hill; winter would come there first, and leave last. The thought made Laurie chilly, and she reached an arm into the mound of bedclothes beside them and pulled a comforter across their bodies. Bill snuggled closer and kissed her twice, gently, on the side of her neck.

Laurie let out a long, luxurious sigh, and closed her eyes. It was a golden moment, a moment to reckon time by, the first such moment in fifteen years of marriage. She worked consciously to memorize the smell of the air, the softness of the sheets, the sound of leaves rustling outside, the exact shade of the soft glow from the nearby street light. Someday she'd want to describe the moment, in all its richness, to her daughter.

The moment had been spontaneous, in a way. No sober discussion had preceded it. Bill would be surprised when she told him, but the ultimate decision had been made months ago, perhaps longer than that, when Laurie had finally admitted to herself, and to Bill, that a career was not enough; she wanted a baby. To Laurie, it had seemed like a one-sided decision. Bill had been ready to start a family for almost as long as they'd been married, and over the years he'd grown less and less subtle about his wish. It had been Laurie who'd always held back. Nor, despite her seeming reticence, had she escaped the baby-craving. Even be-

fore they were married she'd daydreamed about presenting Bill
with a child, a tiny sweet-faced baby wrapped in a blanket. The
fantasy had grown out of a movie she'd seen where June Allyson
had announced to her screen husband that they were going to
have a baby, and then a few scenes later she'd handed him a son.
There had been no tedious pregnancy, no messy labor and delivery, and no eighteen years of child-rearing, only the quintessen-
tial Cinemascope baby fantasy.

She grinned at the thought. Laurie was too much a realist ever
to take such a dream seriously, but, she admitted to herself, that
fantasy had given her a great deal of secret pleasure at one time.
The fantasy changed many times over the years, and the changes
in it mirrored the changes in Laurie. The fantasies grew increasingly realistic, but they never grew strong enough to convince
Laurie that *now* was the time. She had always wanted a baby, but
there had always been reasons, good ones, to wait. It had been
that way right from the beginning. She had, she recalled, thought
a lot about babies after she and Bill first met, when they were
seniors in college, but her thoughts then had all been about how
not to have them.

She had met Bill on the campus tennis courts when she was
paired by chance with him in a mixed-doubles match. Bill was
tall and gangly; he liked to brag that he could play the entire
game from mid-court, his reach was so long. Laurie, on the other
hand, had short, muscular legs and wide hips, but was relatively
slender from the waist up. It was not a physique she would have
picked, had the choice been hers, but it did give her great speed
and maneuverability on the tennis court. They seemed like an
obvious combination for a doubles team.

They lost every game. Laurie insisted on working the back-
court, where her speed would be an advantage, and Bill agreed,
but then refused to trust her and repeatedly lunged to intercept
shots that should have been hers. When the balls got past him,
Laurie was always in position to return them, but by then Bill's
momentum had put him squarely in the way. She hit him with her
shots four times in one game—the first was an accident.

By the end of the match, they were snarling at one another, and only a mutual desire for revenge caused them to agree to play again, singles, a few days later. They never finished that game. Laurie kept Bill running from one edge of the court to the other, and was leading 5–2 when Bill, exhausted, made a dive for a ball, stumbled, landed hard, and badly scraped his right knee. It was late evening, and they were alone on the courts. Laurie helped him up, then helped him limp the several blocks across campus to his small apartment, where she cleaned and bandaged his knee for him.

The animosity vanished in an instant; Laurie had clearly won, but it was not her nature to gloat, nor Bill's to sulk. Instead, Bill offered Laurie his compliments on her tennis game, and a glass of wine, and she accepted both. They sat at Bill's dining table, sipping the wine and talking, but not about tennis. They discussed the upcoming campus elections and then the congressional elections that would be held in November. When they tired of politics they talked about music, and philosophy, and careers. Laurie's major was history and Bill's was accounting; they quickly learned that a common requirement of both disciplines was an eye for minutiae. Now the two of them traded obscure details on pet subjects, and the most frequent remark by either was a surprised "I didn't know that." The conversation, friendly and unforced, went on for hours. When, at two A.M., Bill invited Laurie to spend the night, she declined. He gallantly offered to sleep on the floor, but she said "Don't be silly" and refused, despite earnest arguments from Bill, to let him walk her home.

Bill phoned the next day, and the day after that. They sat together at a movie in the student union, met in the library, strolled across campus together. Bill sent her flowers. That Saturday they rode the bus downtown to attend a matinée concert. On Sunday, they wandered through an art museum. Monday and Tuesday night Laurie stayed home to study for an exam, but Bill phoned both nights and they talked for hours. Wednesday night, Bill took Laurie to dinner at a small Chinese restaurant near his apartment, and afterward they went to the apartment, ostensibly so Laurie could inspect Bill's injured knee. There they drank more wine, and suddenly a touch became a caress, the caress an embrace, the embrace a kiss. The kiss began awkwardly at first, but grew rapidly into a crescendo of passion, and with their arms still around each other they half-walked, half-danced the short distance to Bill's bed.

Neither of them could claim to be particularly surprised; a lot had happened in the eight days since the tennis match. Still, the moment was unplanned, and Laurie was acutely aware of it: Neither she nor Bill had used any birth control. Laurie fretted for three weeks, until her period began, right on schedule. The following week, she went to the campus clinic, where a grandfatherly physician refused to prescribe any sort of birth control without her parents' consent and lectured her gently about the virtues of chastity. She stalked out and went to a private gynecologist, who outfitted her with a diaphragm.

Her relationship with Bill grew—they studied together, played together, fought fiercely on occasion, and seldom spent time with anyone else. By silent agreement, they did not play tennis.

Bill was nearly two years older than Laurie. He had joined the Army at eighteen and had been lucky enough to be sent to Germany instead of Vietnam. He had spent his last few months in the Army at Fort Holabird in Baltimore, and enrolled in college even before he was discharged. His GI benefits, coupled with the money he'd saved in the Army, allowed him to live modestly in an efficiency apartment just across the street from campus.

For Laurie, an only child, college had presented the first opportunity to live somewhere besides home, and she had moved out of her parents' suburban Baltimore house and into a dormitory her freshman year. That year she took her first drink of hard liquor, smoked her first cigarette, and lost her virginity in a highly unsatisfactory fashion at a drive-in movie. She had continued to flirt with all three vices until her grades began to suffer, then substituted coffee for booze and made the dean's list. In the fall of her sophomore year, her roommate left college to get married, and Laurie found that living without a roommate improved her grade average even more. Her steady boyfriend developed an interest in the captain of the women's basketball team and Laurie buried her disappointment in her books. By the end of that year she was eighth in her class. In her junior year she had begun dating a tennis player occasionally, but both were interested more in the game than each other. Laurie stopped dating him when she met Bill.

She continued to live in a dormitory on campus, though she spent many nights at Bill's apartment. The next May, she graduated with honors and, to her parents' utter dismay, moved out of the dorm and into Bill's apartment and began looking for a job. Bill wanted to get a master's degree in business administration and she had announced her intention to support him while he did.

For Bill, who had grown up in a small Kentucky town, that was an uncomfortable proposition. By the standards of his hometown, his views were quite liberal, but he'd never given much thought to the relationship between men and women. Not until he met Laurie, at least. He'd never met a more abrasive, self-centered woman in his life, he thought after their first encounter; he owed it to all malekind to teach her a lesson. Men were natural athletes, and women were not. She ought to learn that. As he had limped back to his apartment after the grudge match, he hadn't rethought his opinions about women in general, only about Laurie. Here was a woman who did not fit the pattern he'd seen all his life: a mother who obeyed his father, an aunt who obeyed his uncle, and on Sundays a fundamentalist preacher who explained from the pulpit why this was necessary. Somehow, Bill knew without asking that Laurie had never been to a fundamentalist church.

When they'd begun to talk, Bill had realized that Laurie was also his equal intellectually, which had made him apprehensive. Smart women, he'd heard, were supposed to be castrating women. Then she'd taken him to bed and shattered even that notion. Except for one or two high-school crushes, Bill had never felt any serious affection for a woman; one day into his relationship with Laurie, Bill was hopelessly in love.

When he decided to go for his MBA, Bill planned to get a part-time job to support himself. He resisted, at first, Laurie's decision to support them. He tried to explain to her that decent men did not live off their women, that he would never take advantage of her in such fashion, that it was his duty to support her, not the other way around.

"Do you think I'm incompetent?" she asked him matter-of-factly.

"You know that's not what I mean," Bill said.

"Lazy?"

"You're missing my whole point. I . . . "

"Greedy, then."

"I'm trying to tell you that it's because I love you!"

"I never thought of that as a disability before."

"Goddammit, Laurie . . . "

"Bill, how long will it take you to finish school if you have to work?"

Bill hung his head, said nothing.

"Two years, right? And how long will it take you to finish if I support us? One year. Now you tell me, which one makes more sense?"

Bill still said nothing. The argument was over, and they both knew it. The next day, Laurie started looking for work. But even in 1967, jobs were scarce for women with honors degrees in history. Laurie applied for a job entitled "junior analyst" at the Department of State and was told that her qualifications were excellent and she would be placed on an eligibility list and notified of the next opening. She never heard anything. She tried all the museums, archives, and historical societies she could locate, and was repeatedly complimented on her excellent academic record but got no job. The college placement office suggested that she take a few education courses and get a teaching certificate. She and Bill began to run out of money.

Reluctantly Laurie answered a want ad and got a secretarial job in a small law office. Her starting salary was sixty dollars a week. In spite of herself, Laurie enjoyed the job. She had been disappointed at having to take a job so unrelated to her field of interest, but as the months passed she began to find a similarity between the legal prose she typed and the history books she loved to read. Both dwelt heavily on events past, and both seemed designed to compare the way things were with the way things ought to be. She began reading the legal documents more closely and one day she spotted a potentially disastrous mistake in one. She pointed it out to her boss, who gratefully corrected the mistake and raised her salary to sixty-five dollars a week. She was thrilled beyond words; that night, she insisted on taking Bill to dinner at "their" Chinese restaurant, where she spent the entire first week's raise and more.

Later they remembered it as a wonderful year. Bill took an impossible course load, studied night and day, and passed everything. In addition he tried, after a fashion, to cook and clean house. He proved to be an excellent cook but a terrible housekeeper; Laurie tidied up the place on weekends. They talked in theoretical terms about children, but always agreed that it would be out of the question to start a family without first getting married.

The next May, Bill received his MBA. In June, he and Laurie were married. It was a no-nonsense ceremony with a small reception afterward at Laurie's parents' house. At the reception, Laurie's father handed her a check for a breathtaking sum of money which, he said, was what he would have spent on a big wedding. Laurie spent part of the money to finance an off-season honeymoon in the Caribbean and the rest to buy a used Mustang. She'd ridden the bus to work for a year and had hated it.

In August, Bill got a job as a "management trainee" with a large insurance company, at a starting salary of one hundred seventy-five dollars a week. Suddenly they were earning a thousand dollars a month between them. They moved to a spacious downtown apartment with wall-to-wall carpeting, air conditioning, and a kitchen with a dishwasher and garbage disposal.

Their roles began to shift subtly. Before, Laurie had been the breadwinner. She had done complex, tedious work, and had done it well, and after a year she was earning seventy-five dollars a week. Bill, with no work experience, was starting out at more than twice that. She told herself that the difference was the MBA, but something in her refused to believe it. Moreover, although she was still doing the same work, she now found herself a housewife as well. Bill worked long days and came home exhausted, in no mood to cook. They began eating in restaurants or bringing home Chinese food. Laurie unenthusiastically learned to broil steaks and kept a supply of them in the refrigerator.

They talked about starting a family. Bill fantasized aloud about having a son to take to baseball games and to go squirrel hunting with in Kentucky. Laurie said that would be fine, but *she* wanted to have a daughter. They agreed that one of each would be appropriate, but not just now. Not until they could afford a house, and not as long as Bill had to travel so much.

Bill's insurance company invested its policyholders' money in apartments and office buildings and businesses, and it protected its investments by sending people like Bill out to make sure the operations were well-run and profitable. The increasingly frequent trips took Bill out of town for two or three days. Laurie was almost grateful for the time alone, because it meant she could read. When Bill was around, they talked, or played, or fought, or made love, or watched television, but always together. They even took baths together.

She never had time to read anymore, and she found it a little frustrating. She had always loved to read, had always read anything and everything within reach. She could lose herself completely in even the dullest history book, reading with a fierce concentration that kept her immobile until aching muscles or a desperately full bladder forced her to put the book aside. Reading too was the only thing that could keep her from smoking for any length of time.

It sometimes seemed to her that her love of reading made Bill jealous; when she tried to read in his presence, he would grow restless and try to talk to her. His words would wrench her mind away from the book and force it to refocus on him, and often that instant of disorientation would sharpen into annoyance, and they would exchange harsh words. After a while, Laurie quit trying to read when he was around.

So, unlike many newlyweds, Laurie cherished her time alone. Typically, she would drive Bill to the airport on Sunday evenings, and Sunday night she would read half a book. Monday evening she would finish that book and begin another, and Tuesday yet another. Bill usually returned on Wednesdays; but he often fell asleep, exhausted, soon after dinner, and Laurie would finish the third book.

Bill had once described Laurie's reading as an addiction worse than heroin, and there were times when Laurie was inclined to agree. Her thirst for the printed word seemed insatiable and, moreover, her retention of detail was almost inhuman. She actually *remembered* that James Madison, at five feet two, was the shortest U.S. President, that an Italian sonnet consisted of four quatrains and a couplet, and that the melting point of titanium was 1668 degrees Centigrade. She used words like "sisyphusian" in ordinary conversation. Bill joked that if they ever got divorced, he would demand an encyclopedia and a dictionary as part of the settlement. Laurie was both flattered and a little bemused by the kidding. She saw nothing unusual in the fact that she enjoyed reading and if she happened to remember the things she read, it was useful. It made her an above-average legal secretary.

She brought home her first law book after her boss had asked her to look up and photocopy a particular Supreme Court case, and before she had finished she became absorbed in reading the case itself. She had been typing quotes from such cases for more than a year, but she'd seldom stopped to think about what she was doing. Now, as she examined the copy of the first page to make sure it was legible, her eye was drawn to the introductory comments at the top of the document, and as she read, a sudden realization burst upon her: *This was history.* More, it was the genuine article, the original source, not someone's interpretation of it. These were the *actual words* that Justice Hugo Black had written for a unanimous Supreme Court. Reading the case was, in a sense, the equivalent of visiting King Tut's tomb, or standing inside Stonehenge at summer solstice, or reading Lincoln's personal letters in the National Archives. This was the real thing. The greatness of humankind lies in its ability to make—and be thrilled by—great discoveries. Archimedes, when he discovered the principle of buoyancy, leaped from his bath and ran naked through the streets shouting "Eureka! Eureka!" Laurie was no less thrilled to discover the first principle of the law, but her only reaction was an overwhelming desire to read the case in front of her. Her boss found her at the copying machine, lost in the book. She blushed and apologized; the lawyer looked at her thoughtfully, and later that day gave her a textbook full of similar cases to take home.

Laurie was quickly hooked. Law, she realized, was simply a mechanism for solving problems, and the fuel for that mechanism was history. No problem need be solved more than once; the solutions were carefully written down and indexed and could be invoked with great weight the next time a similar problem arose. There was even a companion benefit. Laurie, a fast reader, used up a lot of books on her reading binges. It had always seemed faintly wasteful to her. The dense, ponderous prose of law books slowed her down and there was so much of it that, for the first time in as long as she could remember, she took a respectable amount of time to finish a book. She spent two entire weekends on the first book, a weighty collection of cases about personal injury and civil liability. She traded that for one about contracts, then the federal courts, then the rules of evidence.

When her boss suggested she take the Law School Aptitude Test, she hesitated. She was having a wonderful time reading the books, but only because they opened up vast new oceans of trivia for her. She loved the knowledge for its own sweet sake, not because she ever expected to *do* anything with it. She talked it over with Bill, and it was settled. "For all the same reasons you gave for putting me through graduate school, I am going to put you through law school," he said flatly. Laurie took the LSAT and, to no one's surprise, scored in the top four percent. She applied to five law schools including Harvard and Yale and was accepted at all five. Bill's job, however, was in Baltimore, so that fall she quit her secretarial job and enrolled at the University of Maryland School of Law.

The school's rules made it impossible to graduate in less than two-and-a-half years; otherwise Laurie would have done it in two. The bulk of the work was reading, and being able to read, all day and all night if she wanted to, was to Laurie a luxury of almost sinful proportions. Writing and speaking were also required, and Laurie enjoyed neither of those; she did them both slowly and carefully, and relied on her encyclopedic memory to keep her out of trouble. She graduated sixth in her class and got job offers from several of the major law firms.

She turned them all down in favor of a two-year hitch as a junior prosecutor in the state criminal courts. There, in the rough-and-tumble atmosphere of a gigantic justice mill, she learned how to think and talk fast on her feet, learned how to bargain with equally fast-talking defense attorneys, learned when to bluff and when to give up. The hours and the pay were terrible; the education was beyond price. At the end of two years she went back to the same small law firm where she'd worked as a secretary. But now, at age twenty-nine, she was a full partner. The following year, she earned more money than Bill. For almost a decade she and Bill pursued their careers. Bill got an important promotion and once again earned more than Laurie; three years later, as the law firm expanded, Laurie passed him again.

Neither Laurie nor Bill was gregarious by nature, and their circle of friends tended to consist of a few couples their own age. In the early years of their relationship, those friends had been college classmates. There were three other couples with whom they regularly socialized. Then, one by one, the women became pregnant and suddenly Laurie found barriers between her and them. The women no longer wanted to talk about politics, or movies, or anything except what it felt like to be pregnant. And after the babies were born, the disease infected the husbands too, so that their evenings were spent goo-gooing at the baby and talking about when he had first lifted his head and when she'd get her first tooth.

Gradually, they drifted apart from their college friends and met more and more with people from Laurie's law firm or Bill's insurance company. Hardly a week went by without a cocktail party or a backyard barbecue at someone's house, where it was possible to socialize with people whose good will was essential to career advancement. Both Laurie and Bill were younger than most of their colleagues, which meant that in social gatherings they tended to hear more than their share of old war stories and receive more than their share of good advice. Bill tolerated it out of a sense of duty; Laurie, always the historian, claimed to enjoy the war stories.

Their circle of close friends remained small. Laurie's former boss and mentor, now her senior partner, often came to dinner. His wife, a buyer for a large department-store chain, came with him whenever she was in town. One of Bill's fellow junior executives, Jim Walker, shared Bill's taste for the outdoor life. He and his wife, Robbie, and Bill and Laurie took a couple wilderness excursions together, but Laurie and Robbie quickly decided they preferred to vacation in places where bathtubs were nearby, and the camping trips stopped. Once or twice a year, the four of them would catch a Metroliner to New York for an expensive weekend of restaurants and shows. Bill and his friend went fishing together occasionally, and when they did, Laurie always seized the chance to catch up on her reading, since Bill didn't travel much anymore.

They bought a very old house in a very old suburb north of town and invested a great deal of time and money to refurbish it. Bill took up woodworking as a hobby while Laurie bought books on interior decorating. When the house was finished, they began entertaining. Bill's cooking flourished in the spacious new kitchen, and it became Laurie's job to entertain guests while Bill prepared and served dinner. The role reversal amused both of them, and Bill's gourmet meals always drew high praise from their company.

When they both began to gain weight, Bill suggested, somewhat timidly, that they play a game or two of tennis. To their mutual surprise, they had fun and started to play regularly. Neither of them ever suggested that they try doubles.

They started to talk seriously about having babies.

The topic had come up in the past, many times; indeed, Laurie's mother as well as Bill's had been hinting about grandchildren almost since the couple had gotten married. Laurie and Bill had agreed that it would be a good thing to have children, but there had been excuses: law school, the prosecutor's office, the house, and besides, there was still time. Now Laurie was thirty-seven, and Bill began to worry aloud that time was running out. Laurie consulted her gynecologist, who assured her that she was in excellent health and still capable of bearing children.

Bill suggested that she stop using her diaphragm immediately. She agonized, waffled, stalled. Life without children was easy and self-indulgent, and she wasn't at all sure she wanted to change that. After all, no decision was not really a negative decision. But the baby-craving was there and it nagged at her.

Bill wanted children very badly. He had achieved financial and social success beyond anything he'd ever dreamed, and he took great pleasure in inviting his Kentucky relatives to visit so he could show off. Bill's brothers, one a machine-shop foreman, the other a car salesman, had been duly impressed. But they both brought well-behaved adolescent sons with them, and it was Bill who found himself being envious. Bill found many occasions to mention it to Laurie. They discussed and rediscussed the issue of whether they wanted children at all. Raising a family had its drawbacks, after all: There would be no more lazy Saturday mornings, no more impromptu trips to New York. Instead there would be diapers and formula, baby clothes and doctor bills, and probably even the PTA someday. They would be close to sixty years old by the time the child was grown.

There were, they agreed, many good, rational reasons to remain childless. So why, came the inevitable question, were they talking about having children? "Because we want to," Bill would say quietly. "Because there's something missing. I make more money than I ever dreamed of making, and I've got nobody to spend it on."

Laurie put on her best innocent face and pointed a finger toward her chest.

"Hell with that," Bill said, smiling. "You make more than I do. I mean kids. I can give a kid a better start in life than I had, except I don't have any kids."

"You will," Laurie said. "You will. Just don't rush me."

Bill accepted Laurie's reticence with fairly good grace. After all, she seemed genuinely intent on having children, but she also seemed somehow . . . afraid. Stage fright, of a sort, Bill figured. For a time, he considered tampering with her diaphragm, but it was not his nature to be devious or impatient. He was ready whenever Laurie was; he told her that regularly.

On impulse, Laurie phoned one of her college friends who, she knew, had just had a third child. The woman, like Laurie, was thirty-seven. They chatted over coffee, and the woman told Laurie she'd deliberately gotten pregnant again when the first two children reached school age, because she found she missed having an infant to mother. The pregnancy and delivery had been uncomplicated—"Wonderful," Laurie's friend said.

When it was time to pick up the two children at school, the woman deputized Laurie to stay at the house and watch the two-month-old daughter, who at the moment was asleep. No sooner had the mother's car left the driveway than the baby woke and began to cry. Laurie looked around desperately for a bottle, found several, and realized she had no idea what to give the baby. Finally, in desperation, she unbuttoned her blouse, unhooked her bra, and held the baby against her breast.

She would never forget the feeling that came over her as the infant instinctively located her nipple and began nursing. It was a curiously sexual feeling, but not erotic; more sensual, a sort of warm, postorgasmic glow. Laurie worried that the baby would realize she was getting no milk and begin to cry again, but the baby continued to nurse, apparently content with the homegrown pacifier. After a while, the baby grew quiet, her head lolled back, and Laurie replaced her in the crib. When her friend returned, Laurie made excuses and left, and as she drove back to her office, she fantasized about having her own child to breastfeed.

But whatever descriptive terms applied to Laurie, "hasty" was not one of them. The conviction that she wanted a child, wanted one *now,* grew stronger, but Laurie thought about it carefully for several more weeks and continued to be as cautious as ever. The diaphragm she'd gotten in college was the first of a long line of them; it wasn't as absolutely reliable as the pill, but Laurie had a fierce distrust of pills of all sorts and a diaphragm, carefully used, could be very effective indeed.

Laurie was careful. She always used twice as much of the spermicidal gel as was recommended, and she always made extra sure the thing was positioned in exactly the right spot. It was an inconvenience to jump out of bed and visit the bathroom every time, just when the foreplay was about to escalate to lovemaking, but after fifteen years, the routine was so well established that she and Bill hardly noticed it.

Outside, the breeze shifted direction and the expressway sounds were muffled by rustling noises, as the pile of leaves below the bedroom window rearranged itself. Laurie shifted in the bed, sighed, and rolled over, fluffing the pillow and rearranging it under her head. Beside her, Bill snored quietly. Only an hour earlier, she'd jumped out of bed, like always, and had gone into the bathroom and shut the door. She'd taken the diaphragm out of its purple plastic case, had smeared it with gel . . . and then had paused. She'd held the thing at arm's length and studied it for a moment. Then she'd dropped it into the trashcan, tossed the tube of spermicide in after it, and had gone back into the bedroom.

So now, she thought sleepily, she was going to have a baby. A girl, she decided. She wanted a girl. Most certainly she would want to breastfeed the baby. There were a lot of details she'd have to work out. Tomorrow she'd have to start a list.

[2]
Getting Pregnant

THE NEXT DAY Laurie phoned her gynecologist. She hated the gynecological exam, but now was not a time to be squeamish. If she was going to have a baby, she had concluded, she ought first to make sure all the necessary equipment was in good working order. She negotiated with the doctor's secretary and finally agreed on a date two weeks away, which would be just past the end of her next menstrual period, if she had one. If she was late, the secretary said, the doctor would want to check her anyway.

That night, over dinner, she broke the news to Bill. "I've stopped using the diaphraghm," she said without fanfare. "I want to try to get pregnant."

Bill nodded soberly, but said nothing. Instead, he pushed his chair back from the table, stood, and held the back of Laurie's chair. Laurie, thinking he wanted to hug her, stood up. But Bill took her hand and led her out of the kitchen and across the hall to the guest bedroom where he began to remove her clothes.

"Bill, for Chrissake, I'm not finished with dinner yet," Laurie protested. Bill said nothing, removed only the necessary amount of clothing, then lifted Laurie onto the guest bed and made love to her without even a pretense of foreplay. Afterward, she called him an animal.

He grinned down at her. "Naaah," he said confidently. "Neanderthal, maybe, but not animal. An animal would've done it in the kitchen."

"And a gentleman would've asked if I was in the mood," she said pouting.

Bill's face grew serious. "I didn't want to give you a chance to change your mind," he said. "Besides, this is the first time in—'' he did a mental calculation ''—sixteen years that I haven't had to wait for you to put in that goddam diaphragm. How could I resist that kind of temptation?''

Laurie chuckled in spite of herself. It was almost impossible to be irritated at Bill. ''Well, in your own Neanderthal way, I guess you just told me you liked the idea.''

''Like it? *Like* it? Wanna do it again?'' Bill asked.

''Now you're bragging,'' Laurie said, then quickly held up a hand as he moved toward her. ''Okay, okay, you're not bragging. Let me finish dinner first, please?''

They made love again that night, and the next night, and the night after that, and the change in their accustomed routine made it fresh and exciting for both of them. She should have done this long ago, she mused contentedly.

A week later, her period started right on time. She was both disappointed and relieved.

Laurie arrived at the gynecologist's office precisely on time and sat down on a hard plastic chair in the waiting room. She was never late for an appointment, nor was she ever early. The punctuality gave her a sense of being at least partly in control, of being more of a participant and less of a specimen.

She always dreaded these visits, anticipating with a mixture of fear and revulsion the probing, the touching, the cold, clinical, impersonal, emotionless handling. It was an invasion of privacy, she finally decided, resorting to a lawyer's phrase. She looked around the waiting room. There were half a dozen other women seated there, and one was wearing a maternity dress. No one spoke to anyone else. The women read, or fidgeted, or glanced furtively at the other women's hands, checking for rings. Laurie sat stiffly, her face impassive.

As always, the doctor was behind schedule. Laurie tried to feel superior, and it didn't work. She tried thinking about her job, and that didn't work either. She thought about the last play she'd attended, the last symphony, the last vacation in the Caribbean, but nothing worked. Her stomach continued to flutter, and a tiny wisp of panic darted around the edges of her consciousness. How she hated these exams!

She had spent nearly half an hour in the shower that morning, lathering repeatedly. Afterward she had applied powder and deodorant, but there is no antiperspirant that can stop nervous sweat. By the time the nurse called her name she could already feel the clamminess.

She followed the nurse into an examining room, accepted a folded paper gown, and watched the nurse leave. She glanced around the room, examining the sink, the clothing stand, the supply cabinet, the small stool, the little stainless-steel wastebasket on wheels, and the waist-high examining table with the gleaming metal stirrups at one end. Slowly, she undressed. As always, she had worn conservative and immaculately clean cotton underwear. As always, she folded it neatly, put it on the chair beside the clothing stand, then folded her skirt and blouse and laid them on top of the underwear.

She stood a moment, naked, and debated throwing the ridiculous paper gown into the little rolling trashcan. Without the gown she would merely be nude; wearing it, she was worse than naked, she was helpless, a ludicrous piece of half-draped cheesecake. She'd be tacitly accepting *their* rules, surrendering her dignity without a fight. But this was not, she reminded herself, an adversary proceeding. She was here voluntarily; hell, she was *paying* for this. Sighing, she tied the gown around her, hoisted herself onto the table, and sat grimly, palms on the table, waiting.

The room was a trifle chilly, so that when a drop of icy perspiration trickled down her ribs, she stirred and dabbed at it with the paper gown. The nurse came back in and took her blood pressure. Laurie submitted without a word, wondering angrily why it was necessary for her to undress *before* they took her blood pressure. The nurse unwrapped the blood pressure cuff, instructed Laurie to lie down on the table, helped her fit her heels into the steel stirrups, and left. Laurie lay there, her back sticking to the waxed-paper sheet on the table, and tried to relax. Sooner than she expected, the nurse and doctor walked into the room.

The doctor's questions were to the point. Laurie answered in monosyllables. She tensed when the doctor touched her, forced herself to relax. She tried to remind herself of the benefits of the examination, and instead found herself hoping he wouldn't be so thorough that he'd notice her underarms were soaking wet. The doctor straightened, moved toward the end of the table. "Okay, scoot down a bit, please," he said. "More. A little more. That's it, a little more. Fine."

The paper gown blocked her view, but she heard a *click* as the doctor switched on the goose-neck lamp, and she felt the warmth of the lamp as he drew it close to her. She heard a drawer of the cabinet slide open, and then the stool scraped across the floor and the trashcan banged against the side of the examining table. Laurie breathed deeply and regularly, her teeth clenched. She couldn't see the doctor now, and she flinched when his hands touched her knees, gently forcing them apart.

The speculum was warm to the touch. She felt a slight stretching sensation as the device opened. She tried to estimate its size, but could not. She heard a brief clatter of instruments, and then felt a tiny pressure somewhere inside, almost unnoticeable. Then she felt the speculum being released and withdrawn.

She tensed again when she felt the doctor's fingers enter her and she tried to relax. Now there was pressure and it was uncomfortable, but it wasn't painful, and it was for her benefit. Her benefit. Her benefit . . .

Abruptly the pressure ceased, and she heard the rubber glove snap as the doctor pulled it off and dropped it into the rolling trashcan. She let out a long, quiet breath as she heard the stool scrape across the floor. The nurse helped her out of the stirrups, handed her a wad of tissue, and left her alone. The perspiration stopped, leaving Laurie feeling chilly and unclean. She dressed, and spent an uncharacteristically long time adjusting her hair.

In the gynecologist's office, Laurie demanded to know why she hadn't gotten pregnant. The gynecologist looked pained. "I'd be more surprised if you had," he answered carefully. "Most people have to try for a while. Out of every hundred women actively trying to get pregnant, sixty of them will succeed within a year."

"I can't afford to wait a year, can I?" she asked.

The doctor paused. "A year, sure," he said, finally. "Two years, three years—it's hard to say. You're in better condition than most thiry-seven-year-old women I see, and that makes a difference, too.

"Let me put it this way: I can't find any reason to tell you *not* to get pregnant. There are risks, both for you and for the baby, and they increase as you get older, but right now, and for the next couple of years, those risks are comparatively few, less than five percent."

"What sort of risks?" Laurie asked, leaning slightly forward. She fought an impulse to take notes.

"For you, diabetes. High blood pressure. Less likely, but possible, premature labor. Those are the most common. There are other things, like a certain form of cancer that prefers pregnant women, but those are extremely rare.

"Obviously, those things are also a risk for the baby. Then there's the risk of Down's syndrome. It used to be called mongolism. You know what that is."

Laurie nodded. "And the risk of all that is five percent right now," she said.

"Probably a little less than that right now," the doctor replied. "It's all age-related, and you're a very young thirty-seven. Don't lose your perspective. There's a slight risk, to be sure, but there's a much greater chance that everything will be fine.

"However," he went on, "there is the little matter of your smoking." Laurie's eyes fell. "If you smoke during pregnancy, you'll have a smaller baby. That's the only proven effect, but there is some evidence to suggest that you will also have a less intelligent baby.

"There is your blood pressure, which is a little bit elevated this time. Quitting smoking might help that, too. I know I tell you that every time you come in here, but this time I really mean it. You really should quit."

"You're right," Laurie replied, "I really should, and I'll try, but I make no promises."

The conversation concluded with pleasantries, and Laurie left to go to work. But on the way, she went home and took another shower.

The following afternoon, while looking up a court case in the firm's small library, she reached for a cigarette and discovered her pack was empty. It was an omen, she decided; the gods were telling her that it was time to quit smoking. She located the law book she wanted, sat down in a hard-backed chair, and tried to read. Presently one of the firm's other lawyers walked in, watched Laurie fidget awhile, then observed aloud that Laurie must be trying to quit smoking.

"It's that obvious, huh?" she asked ruefully. Her partner agreed. When he had quit smoking, he said, he had found it useful to take deep breaths every time he felt the nicotine craving. It made him feel healthier, he said, and eventually he came to equate the nicotine craving with a feeling of good health. It was all a matter of training the subconscious, he said. Laurie agreed politely, and took several deep breaths at the partner's urging.

The craving did not go away; it got worse. Laurie had smoked cigarettes, and enjoyed them thoroughly, for nearly twenty years; the nicotine fit she was experiencing now blended two decades of addiction with the fact that she didn't really *want* to quit. She riffled through the case book several times, then read the same page three times without absorbing a word. Finally, in desperation, she took a dozen huge breaths and got spots in front of her eyes. The craving persisted.

She left work early, and on the way home she stopped at a convenience store and bought a carton of cigarettes. She'd quit as soon as she got pregnant, she promised herself as she lit the first one.

Her period started right on schedule the next month and the following one. She was three days late the month after that, and was profoundly disappointed when it did start. Then back on schedule, twenty-eight days, twenty-eight days, twenty-eight days. Laurie celebrated her thirty-eighth birthday. Her periods continued to come regularly, right on time. She phoned the gynecologist.

"Don't try so hard," he told her. "I can tell you stories about couples that tried for years, and when they finally gave up and adopted a child, the woman got pregnant. Forget you're trying to get pregnant. Surprise yourself." That was easy for *him* to say, Laurie thought as she hung up the phone.

She called her friend with the three children. They had a long lunch at a restaurant overlooking the harbor, drank white wine, and exchanged gossip about other classmates. Finally Laurie confided that she was trying to get pregnant and not succeeding. Her friend looked sympathetic. "Have you tried standing on your head?" she asked.

Laurie stared. "Have I tried what?"

"You know, afterwards," the friend said, blushing. "Think about it. Those little things have to swim upstream. If you stand on your head, they'll be swimming downstream instead, and you'll make it easier for them. More of them will get where they need to go."

Laurie thought about it. She tried it once, for about a minute. Bill started snickering and humming "Row, row, row your boat, gently down the stream." Laurie started laughing, and lost her balance. Then she tried lying on her back with her heels propped against the wall, but by then it was impossible to be serious about it, so instead they made love again. Trying to have a baby had certainly improved their sex life, Laurie reflected. Bill had performed faithfully—relentlessly, it seemed sometimes.

In fact, Bill's performance was motivated more by fear than desire. He had reached the point in life where he'd begun to wonder why he worked so hard to earn so much money if he had no children to leave it to. Now, at least, Laurie was willing to have babies and he seemed unable to impregnate her. After the third month, he'd secretly visited his own doctor and masturbated into a test tube to find out if he was fertile. He was. His doctor gave him the same advice as Laurie's: Relax and keep trying.

At her gynecologist's suggestion, Laurie began keeping a temperature chart. On the day the chart predicted maximum fertility, she and Bill made love in the morning and again that night. Ten days later her period started, right on schedule. Laurie and Bill spent a gloomy night in front of the fireplace, got very drunk, and talked, for the first time, about adopting a child.

The following month, Bill showed up unannounced at her office and suggested a nooner for good luck, but Laurie scowled and chased him out. She had a new case to worry about, and suddenly she had no time to think about getting pregnant.

It was an unusual suit. The divorce court had awarded custody of two small girls, aged five and seven, to their father, an assistant manager in a supermarket. It had come out during the hearing that the mother, a nurse, had a violent temper, and had hit the children, in front of witnesses, on several occasions. The judge had based his custody ruling on that testimony and had disregarded the recommendation of the child welfare department, which had suggested, as it always did, that the mother be given custody. Now the mother was appealing the decision. The father had been represented by one of the junior associates in Laurie's law firm. Laurie was brought into the case, both because she handled nearly all the firm's appellate work and because the partners felt there was a tactical advantage to having the father represented by a woman.

Laurie had never handled a child-custody matter of any sort, so she buried herself in case books. She read them in her spare time at the office and took books home with her at night. The temperature charts became an unwelcome distraction, and she abandoned them. She met with the father, then arranged to visit his house one evening to meet his daughters. She read and reread the transcript of the divorce hearing and the child-welfare caseworker's report. Most important, she read the formal opinions that had been issued in all the other, similar cases she could find.

There were a number of appeals on the ground that a judge

should give more weight to the social worker's report than had been given in this particular case. After a few days of research Laurie had found an equally impressive list of decisions in which the judge was given a great deal of discretion in such matters. She fashioned her argument around these cases, smiling to herself: Just beneath the surface, her argument was saying that judges were strong and learned men capable of making tough decisions. It was an argument calculated to make a good impression on a panel of judges.

In an appellate hearing, oral arguments are a verbal rough-and-tumble between the attorneys and the judges over the fine technicalities and grand theories of the particular case. Oral arguments rarely change the judges' minds, but they often give attorneys a hint of which side will prevail. Laurie got more than hints. The three judges lured the other lawyer far out onto a theoretical limb, then set upon him with a vengeance and picked his argument to shreds. When Laurie argued, though, the judges were all smiles and tacitly agreed that yes, judges *were* strong and learned men. Tradition forbade them to decide the matter on the spot, but when Laurie walked out of the courtroom she knew she'd won.

It had been a frustrating time for Bill; Laurie had ignored him for the better part of a month. That night, Laurie took Bill to his favorite restaurant for an early dinner, then to the new symphony hall for a concert. Afterward they stopped at a bar and got tipsy on cognac, then drove home and drank more cognac, and finally toppled into bed and made love for the first time in weeks. They awoke hung over and horny, and found that making love actually helped the hangovers. They both got to work late.

Three weeks later, Laurie realized she was pregnant.

Her period was only three days late, which had happened before, but she *knew*, somehow, that this was not a drill. She called her gynecologist's office and arranged for a blood test. Three days later the doctor himself phoned her at work. "Congratulations," he said without fanfare.

Laurie fought back the emotion, forced herself to remain analytical. "I am thirty-eight years old now," she said crisply, "and

I'll be thirty-nine when the baby's born. Let's talk about the risks one more time." As she spoke, she stubbed out a half-smoked cigarette, reached into her purse, and threw the unfinished pack into the trashcan. A vow was, after all, a vow. She took a deep breath and tried to concentrate on the gynecologist's words.

"Technically, you're a high-risk patient because of your age, but what that really means is that instead of having a ninety-seven percent chance for a successful pregnancy, you've got a ninety-four or ninety-five percent chance. You can improve those odds by seeing a high-risk specialist, but the odds are pretty damn good in any case."

Like a good lawyer, Laurie had prepared her next question well in advance. "If I were your wife," she said slowly, "who would you send me to?"

The doctor didn't hesitate. "To the same person I was about to recommend anyway. To Dr. Crenshaw at the University of Maryland."

[3]

Dr. Carlyle Crenshaw

COMPARED TO the average depart-
ment chairman's office, Carlyle Crenshaw's office is modest, almost spartan. Doctors and professors at the top of the academic
heap often celebrate their accomplishments by appropriating a
suite of rooms and outfitting it, usually at their own expense,
with large wooden desks, comfortable furniture, and signed lith-
ographs on the walls.

The desk Carlyle Crenshaw uses is state issue, made of sheet
metal and formica. So is his credenza, and his chair, and the
other odd bits of furniture crowded into a room that looks as
though it was built to contain a hospital bed. Visitors to Crenshaw's office see little of the furniture, though; every square inch
of surface, including a good bit of floor, is stacked with journals
to read, papers to review, letters to answer, medical records to fill
out, inquiries to respond to, applications to consider, and innu-
merable other things to do.

If he thought about it, Crenshaw might well conclude that a
spacious office with fine furniture would be nice, and indeed
someday he may have one, but for the moment he has higher
priorities. He came to the University of Maryland in 1980, with a
mandate from the university to turn its neglected and failing obstetrics program into a world-class operation. By all estimates he
has done just that, but it has left him little time to think about
furniture.

To be ranked with the finest, an academic medical program
must do several things. It must provide the finest medical care—
doctors call it "tertiary" or third-level care—available anywhere. That requires the best doctors you can find, and the most
sophisticated diagnostic machinery you can buy. Crenshaw
spends a lot of time looking for both.

To be truly world-class, though, you must also shine academically. You must do research, important research; you must make significant contributions to scientific and medical knowledge. And you must train new doctors so thoroughly and so brilliantly that when, in a few years, their careers begin to skyrocket, word will get around that they trained at the University of Maryland.

Given a choice, Crenshaw would spend more time on research and teaching, but increasingly, he delegates that job to others, so he can concentrate on the most important job of all: politicking. The cost of health care is front-page news, and teaching hospitals, which are the most expensive of all, are under the greatest pressure to cut back. You cannot run a world-class obstetrics and gynecology program without resources, so Crenshaw spends more and more of his time cruising the centers of academic power, shaking hands and making friends, gathering the support he knows he will need at budget time. That, in turn, gets him appointed to a disproportionate number of boards, committees, commissions, conferences, and ad hoc study groups, all of which are politically useful but time-consuming. Crenshaw comes to work early, leaves late, and carries work home with him every night.

And he sees patients. Despite all the demands on his time, his medical practice remains a priority. Twice a week, he spends half a day in a small suite of private offices down the hall from his departmental office. One day in four he is on call, which for an obstetrician often means no sleep. Sometimes the next day he falls asleep in committee meetings, but he has no thought of giving up the one part of his professional life that, even after thirty years, remains fresh, exciting, and challenging. The cluttered office reflects, without apology, the priorities Carlyle Crenshaw has set for himself and his department.

The phone on Crenshaw's desk buzzed, and he reached for it absently. His eyes remained fixed on the report he was reading. "Yes, ma'am," he said quietly into the receiver.

Just reminding him, the secretary said, that his first appointment was only a couple of minutes away.

"Thank you," he said, eyes still on the report. He hung up the phone, turned one last page, then laid the report down in the center of the cluttered desk. He stubbed out his cigarette, stood and stretched, picked up his coffee cup and headed for the door. The report could wait.

To her amazement, Laurie found an empty parking space on Greene Street, right in front of the main entrance to the hospital. There was even time on the meter.

She had wanted to arrive at Crenshaw's office precisely on time, but had expected to spend time hunting a parking spot. Now, suddenly, she had time to kill. She sat behind the wheel for a long moment, staring up at the great hulking hospital building. She had to lean forward to glimpse the top, thirteen floors up. Red brick and windows, functional and unadorned, stretched away left, right, and up from the corner. The place had eight hundred-odd beds, she recalled reading somewhere. From the look of the building she would have guessed more.

She took a deep breath, then another, and forced herself to concentrate on details of the building's exterior. She had gone to law school near this same complex of buildings, but that had been fifteen years and many new buildings ago. The north wing of the hospital was clearly much newer than the south one; its brick and windows were denser, the lines crisper, the profile more aloof and businesslike. The old wing, halfway down the block, had exposed concrete interspersed with the brick, creating the effect of cornerstones. There was a hint of a portico at the entranceway to the old building; the new entrance was a wall of plate glass doors that opened onto a short covered driveway packed with taxicabs.

It certainly was not the most luxurious-looking hospital she'd seen, Laurie decided, but then, she reminded herself, luxury was not her first consideration. Her gynecologist had been emphatic about that. She glanced at her watch. Twenty minutes to kill. She reached between the car seats and retrieved her purse, checking again to make sure she had the six-page medical history form the secretary had sent her when she'd made the appointment. It was one of those machine-scored forms that had to be filled out with a soft lead pencil, and it had caused Bill to ask whether she was visiting an obstetrician or a computer. With another deep breath, she opened the car door and stepped out. She walked around to the parking meter, dropped quarters to move the arrow up to the two hour limit, then turned and walked the short distance to the hospital entrance.

Laurie paused inside the double glass doors and surveyed the small, inhospitable lobby. On one wall, clerks behind plate glass teller's windows handed out visitor's passes; on the other side, two men in police uniforms stood behind a semicircular desk guarding the passageway to the hospital elevators. In the center of the room there were wooden benches surrounding a large square planter box. There was no other furniture.

Laurie wondered briefly if she would need a pass, and decided to bluff her way through. As she strode briskly across the lobby, she reached into her purse and withdrew her Bar Association identification. She held it up as she walked past the guards, and they smiled and nodded. So much for security, she thought.

Once past the guards, she turned and walked down a long hallway to the old part of the building, and from there she followed her nose to the hospital cafeteria. Inside, there were several different serving lines, but the only crowded one was the cashier's line, which also served coffee and pastries. Laurie looked around; most of the people in the cafeteria were drinking coffee and eating pastries. The line that served hot food had only one customer, a slight, middle-aged man with mussed hair and glasses. As Laurie watched, the cafeteria worker handed him a plate containing two limp pasta shells covered with tomato sauce, and the man carried the tray to the cashier's line. He stood behind Laurie. Two men in scrub suits joined the queue, and Laurie heard one of them say, admiringly, "Oh, look, they're serving placentas again today."

"Oh, my," said the man with the stuffed shells. "Oh, my. Oh, my." Laurie turned around just in time to see the man leave the line, put his tray on a table, and bolt out the cafeteria door.

The men in scrub suits giggled uncontrollably, and Laurie couldn't help but grin. The cafeteria had had a bad reputation when she was in law school, and it clearly had not gotten any better. Laurie drew a large cup of coffee from the shiny urn, paid for it, and sat down at one of the tables. She spent the next ten minutes sipping the coffee and reading over the obstetric questionnaire one more time. Finally, she glanced at her watch, downed the last of the coffee, and started back toward the main elevators.

By her watch, her appointment was three minutes away when she arrived at the elevator lobby. Plenty of time. She stepped back and surveyed the lighted indicators above each set of doors. Of eight elevators, five were on low-numbered floors going up, two were at the first floor going down, and one showed nothing at all. Laurie fiddled with her purse, looked at the elevator lights, inspected a spot on the floor, looked at the elevator lights, read the headlines inside two newspaper boxes, and looked at the elevator lights. Most of the cars were now above the ninth floor, still going up. One was at the sub-basement and its "up" indicator was lighted; another was at the basement level, still going down.

A man standing next to Laurie lit a cigarette. Laurie smelled the smoke and moved away. She hadn't had a cigarette for eleven days, and the agony was almost unbearable. She had tried deep breathing, rock candy, worry beads, chewing gum, catnip, patent medicines, meditation, and chanting; nothing had lessened the craving, and only her iron determination had kept her from smoking. Even that, at times, felt precarious. The smell of cigarette smoke was an almost unbearable temptation; if the man carried his cigarette onto the elevator, she decided, she'd wait for another.

Laurie inspected the newspaper headlines again, read the "staff only" sign beside a wall phone, then read the "no smoking" sign beside the elevators, glanced at the man with the cigarette, then looked at the elevator lights. Now two cars were at the sub-basement, showing "up" arrows but not moving, and the others were hovering around twelve and thirteen. Two were starting down.

Casually, Laurie inspected the small crowd that had begun to gather outside the elevator doors. There was an elderly woman in a wheelchair, accompanied by a teenaged girl in a striped uniform. The old woman had a patch over one eye, and an IV bottle hung above the wheelchair. A middle-aged couple in shabby clothes stood with their arms around each other, eyes fixed on the elevator lights. A very young and very pregnant woman in a cheap blue maternity dress leaned against the wall with one shoulder and stared straight ahead with unfocused eyes.

The elevator bell startled Laurie. Inches behind her, the elevator doors swung open and four people, two in white lab coats and two in green scrub suits, got off. Laurie stepped into the car and stood back against the wall, by the control panel, while the rest of the crowd shuffled silently inside. The man with the cigarette didn't get on.

The doors closed, the car moved briefly, then slowed. A deep mechanical voice intoned "second floor." The woman in the wheelchair and her attendant got off. Laurie looked at her watch, then at the elevator controls. Six—the obstetrics floor—was the next button lit. The car stopped at three, four, and five. Two people in lab coats and one in a scrub suit got on. By the time the elevator announced "sixth floor" Laurie was so annoyed at being late that she had forgotten to be nervous.

She had also forgotten the directions the secretary had given her when she'd made the appointment. She stepped off the elevator, stopped and fumbled with her purse until the pregnant woman got off, and watched her as she walked a few steps to what was clearly a waiting room. It had wire-reinforced glass panels in the doors, and rows of blue vinyl airport-style seats inside. The pregnant woman opened the door, spoke briefly to the receptionist inside, then released the door, turned, and trudged off down a long hallway. Laurie could make out a sign that said "Delivery Room" at the far end of the hallway.

Laurie walked to the waiting room door and pulled it open.

Inside were a dozen or so women of every color and description, dressed in clothes that ranged from plain to downright shabby. Laurie suddenly felt awkwardly overdressed in her gray skirt and white ruffled blouse, her standard lawyer's uniform. The receptionist ignored her for a long moment, then looked up. "Yes?"

"Laura Edwards," Laurie said.

The receptionist consulted a list. "Do you have an appointment?" she asked.

"I'm supposed to see Dr. Crenshaw five minutes ago," Laurie answered.

The receptionist's expression changed. "Oh, you're in the wrong waiting room. Private patients are down the hall," she said, pointing. "There's a sign on the door."

The private offices had green carpeting and soft lights, and modern furniture. On several walls were oriental-style paintings of flowers by an artist whose name Laurie didn't recognize. At the wood-paneled reception desk, a nurse handed Laurie a blue one-page form asking for insurance information, and when she had filled that out, the nurse escorted her down a hallway to a tiny room, where she took Laurie's blood pressure, weighed her, and measured her height. Then the nurse showed her to a small bathroom and handed her a paper cup with her name written on it.

There is no delicate way for a woman to collect a urine specimen, Laurie thought as she removed her skirt, peeled down her pantyhose and sat on the toilet. She maneuvered the cup into position, strained briefly, and peed on her fingers. She cursed, moved the cup, caught a specimen, put the dripping cup on a shelf above the sink, and reached for the toilet paper.

At least, she reflected darkly as she washed her hands, they'd taken her blood pressure while she had her clothes on. Be grateful for small favors.

She left the specimen on the shelf as instructed and walked down a series of corridors back to the waiting area. There were comfortable couches and chairs, and only one other patient was waiting.

In only a few minutes, one of the doors opened and a stocky man with gray hair and half-moon glasses walked out, inspected the charts in the rack beside the door, lifted one out and, reading from the label, said "Mrs. Edwards?"

The doctor waited at the door while Laurie walked the short distance, then held out his hand. "I'm Dr. Crenshaw," he said in a soft Southern baritone. "Come in and sit down."

The first few minutes were occupied with pleasantries. Crenshaw said nice things about Laurie's gynecologist, and Laurie answered that the man had spoken highly of Crenshaw. They discovered a mutual love of Scotland. Laurie and Bill had visited there twice; Crenshaw had friends there. He said he never refused in invitation to lecture at Edinburgh.

In fact, he said, seizing on the topic of travel, he ought to explain right away that he might not always be the doctor who would see her. Within the obstetrics department, he explained, was a team of high-risk specialists who had formed a group practice. They rotated on-call duty and covered for each other during the inevitable interruptions of academic life. All the doctors in the group were faculty members in the medical school's department of obstetrics and gynecology.

"I have to brag a little," Crenshaw said. "Our facilities aren't what they should be here, but we've got some really good people."

For one, he said, he had Dr. David Nagey. Dr. Nagey was young and brilliant. He'd entered college at fifteen, medical school at eighteen. On his way through med school he'd paused to earn a Ph.D. in engineering. His big thing was mathematical modeling, describing medical events in mathematical terms, which made computer-assisted diagnosis possible.

And then there was Dr. Marcos Pupkin. Dr. Nagey sends his wife to see Dr. Pupkin, Crenshaw said. Dr. Pupkin had trained at the University of Chile in Santiago, and had probably delivered five thousand babies by the time he came to the United States. "He's seen everything at least twice," Crenshaw said, "and knows at least two ways to handle it."

Because of her age, Crenshaw said, Laurie would be considered a high-risk patient and would always see a member of the high-risk team when she came in for her regular appointments.

"I want to talk about those risks," Laurie began, but Crenshaw held up a hand.

"I can give you better answers after I know more about you," he said. "Do you have the form we sent?"

Laurie handed it over, and Crenshaw read through it slowly. The questionnaire had a column of standard inquiries about Laurie's medical history, as well as Bill's and both their families'. Then there was a long list of more specific questions about Laurie.

The form asked if and when she had had rubella, hepatitis, polio, rheumatic fever, syphilis, ulcers, high blood pressure, nervous breakdowns. Laurie had admitted to having an occasional urinary infection, and had answered the rest "no." She had never had surgery, never had a broken bone, and took no drugs regularly. She had no drug allergies that she knew of. She had never had a blood transfusion, drank moderately, and, she had written after a bit of thought, she didn't smoke.

Without looking up from the form, Dr. Crenshaw absently reached into a pocket, withdrew a pack of Kent Super Lights, tapped one out, and lit it with a gold Dunhill lighter. Laurie stared open-mouthed as he took a long, luxurious drag on the cigarette. A doctor who smoked! Part of her was fascinated, part was scandalized, and part wanted desperately to be somewhere, anywhere, else. The smoke wafted toward her, and she squeezed the armrests on her chair, turned her face away, tried not to breathe. Dr. Crenshaw took another puff, still reading the form.

A page-and-a-half of the form was devoted to discussion of Laurie's menstrual cycle. After seeing all the things that could go wrong, Laurie had rather proudly marked the spaces indicating that she was as regular as clockwork, seldom had cramps, had a normal flow lasting three to five days. One question asked if the frequency of her periods had changed at all in the past year, and, remembering the one time she'd been three days late, she had answered "yes." Crenshaw stopped reading and asked for details. Laurie explained.

"Was there anything unusual about that period except that it was late?" he asked.

"No."

"Good." He took another deep drag on the cigarette, jotted a note on the form, and continued reading.

There were even a few questions about her sex life: how often she had intercourse, whether she had orgasms (because of the uterine contractions involved), whether intercourse was ever painful for her. Crenshaw stubbed out his cigarette as he turned over the last page of the questionnaire. Then he looked up. "This looks great," he said. "Let's get you set up so I can examine you now."

The examining room was adjacent to the office, with a connecting door. The first thing Laurie noticed was that the stirrups had white cloth covers over them.

Laurie undressed, wrapped herself in the paper smock and bedsheet, and sat on the table. The connecting door was closed, but she could hear Crenshaw dictating. Presently the voice stopped and Crenshaw, accompanied by a nurse, came into the examining room.

The examination that followed made every other physical she had ever received seem perfunctory. Crenshaw examined her eyes, her ears, her nostrils, and her throat. He pounded her joints with a rubber hammer, felt the pulse in her neck and the glands in her armpits, listened with a stethoscope to her chest, back, and abdomen, and then tapped all the same places with his fingers. Laurie noted that his hands were warm. He examined her breasts uncomfortably thoroughly. He even examined her feet. He drew a blood sample, himself, painlessly. He looked at the blood-pressure reading the nurse had written down earlier, then got out a pressure cuff and read it again himself.

Finally, inevitably, the nurse helped Laurie into the stirrups, and from the other side of the bedsheet Crenshaw encouraged her to move closer to the end of the table. Laurie heard the metal stool scrape across the floor and she gritted her teeth.

[4]

The Examination

THE PELVIC EXAMINATION is the cornerstone of modern obstetrics and gynecology. There is no laboratory test, no electronic imaging device, no computerized questionnaire that can replace it. All those things add to the picture, but what the physician sees with his own eyes and feels with his own hands is the information that he most often acts on. And in an age of scientific medicine the pelvic exam remains an art, a thing that cannot be learned from a book, programmed into a computer, or articulated in the professional literature.

Doctors learn this art on the job, with long, patient practice. The first five you do, the residents like to tell the medical students, are purely social visits; for the next hundred or so, all you can feel is warm-and-wet. After that, if you persevere, if you really pay attention, you may begin to feel something significant.

At age fifty-two, Carlyle Crenshaw had been doing pelvic exams for thirty years or more, ever since his days as a medical student at Duke University. He had seen all the common variations in the female reproductive anatomy and a great number of uncommon ones. He knew what everything should look like, where it should be, how it should feel, when to worry, and, more important, when not to worry. Happily, obstetrics was a business in which most worries proved to be unfounded. That was one of the attractions of the field, but it was not what lured Carlyle Crenshaw in the beginning.

At the Duke Medical Center, Carlyle, like every other medical student, had rotated through the various services. He performed the obligatory operation in the animal lab, listened attentively to heart surgeons and brain surgeons, and never saw one of them crack a smile. Internal medicine was absorbing, the hands-on practice it entailed was illuminating, and everyone called everyone else "doctor." In radiology you could go for days without saying a word to a patient. Radiologists usually talked only to doctors or wrote memoranda to them. So Carlyle was ripe for what happened during the first lecture he attended in obstetrics.

The department chairman himself, a formidable man of national reputation, was addressing the medical students. Carlyle took notes carefully. The professor finished his remarks and invited questions.

"What makes you think you know what the hell you're talking about?" came a voice from the back of the auditorium. Carlyle and his fellow students froze in their seats, waiting for the explosion. To their further amazement, the chairman's reaction was profane delight.

"You no-good sonofabitch," he shouted back. "Who let you in here? C'mere. Get your ass down here." The two men shook hands, embraced, and the chairman introduced the class to a former student of his, now chairman of his own department and an illustrious gynecologist in his own right.

Carlyle was spellbound. Here were two giants in the business joking and swapping insults as though they genuinely enjoyed themselves. And using first names. *First names*! He hadn't heard a first name since he began his rotations. Could it be that there was a medical specialty where informality was permitted? He was hooked. He knew it before he ever left the auditorium. Today, thirty-odd years and many academic triumphs later, his department operates with the same kind of freewheeling informality that he so admired in his own first department chairman.

Dr. Crenshaw's department is one of the country's most highly regarded centers for high-risk obstetrics, and he himself is consistently ranked among the top maternal–fetal-medicine specialists in the country. But what is most important to Carlyle Crenshaw is that he enjoys himself.

As a medical discipline, obstetrics, and even high-risk obstetrics, is always absorbing, often challenging, and usually very rewarding. The odds weigh heavily in favor of a good outcome. Nine times out of ten, everything turns out fine. Nine times out of ten, a woman could never visit a doctor at all and still have a normal, healthy baby. The trick is to identify the tenth one.

By the best scientific screening techniques available today, it is possible to identify only two-thirds of the mothers who will, during their pregnancy, encounter some difficulty that threatens either them or their unborn child. The other third will develop problems unexpectedly, usually suddenly, and often disastrously.

Some mothers, particularly in their later reproductive years, will develop diabetes during a pregnancy; untreated, the disease can kill the baby. Occasionally, it kills the mother as well. Others develop high blood pressure, which can severely retard fetal growth and, worse, can develop into a condition most widely known by its archiac name, toxemia. The word, which means literally "blood poisoning," hearkens to a day when the condition was thought to be a blood disorder. As physicians studied it more closely, they realized it wasn't blood poisoning at all; it was something very strange indeed.

There were two separate, identifiable stages to the condition and the doctors began to distinguish between them by calling them preeclampsia and eclampsia. In preeclampsia, the mother's blood vessels begin constricting, and her blood pressure rises alarmingly. If it is left untreated, the condition will choke off the blood supply to the uterus, killing the fetus a short while before the mother's kidneys burn out or, alternatively, she dies of a massive stroke. When the blood pressure gets so high that it causes seizures, the condition is called eclampsia.

It is possible to identify some at-risk women simply by family history; if two sisters and one grandmother had the same problem, then you know to watch for it. If a woman has high blood pressure to begin with, her danger is greater. But a woman's previous obstetric history is only marginally useful; preeclampsia is most often a disease of first pregnancies.

As Carlyle Crenshaw knows only too well, you can never be sure. So, moments after Laurie vacated the small bathroom at the end of the hallway, a nurse walked in, took the small cup of urine from the shelf, emptied it into a plastic specimen container, labeled it with Laurie's name and patient ID number, and attached a computer slip to route it to the clinical laboratory. There technicians would check it for sugar, which warns of diabetes, and protein, which warns of high blood pressure. And, because no good physician ever blindly trusts another physician's diagnosis, the lab would also assay the urine for human chorionic gonadotropin to make sure Laurie is really pregnant.

Meanwhile, Dr. Crenshaw, pulling on an examining glove, scooted the metal stool up close to the end of the examining table and set about the practice of his art. When it is done by an experienced physician, the pelvic exam provides a mountain of subjective information, and not a little objective data as well. Most important of all is the negative information, the absence of reason to worry, the opportunity to rule out possible problems.

As he adjusted the stool, Crenshaw's eyes swept across Laurie's entire pelvic region, noting the absence of surgical scars, estimating the girth of her hips, appraising the muscular, athletic legs, cataloging the pattern of her pubic hair. Laurie's pubic hair was a small, dark triangle, the classic gynecoid pattern. Most women had that triangular pubic-hair pattern, but a significant number had instead a long, narrow, vertical hair pattern, known as an android pattern. Taken alone, the hair patterns meant nothing; they were merely Nature's choice of decoration for a given individual. But statistically, an android hair pattern coupled with menstrual irregularities was strongly suggestive of certain hormone imbalances that could cause infertility. Before he had finished adjusting the stool, Crenshaw had collected enough data to know he probably wouldn't have to worry about Laurie's hormonal balances.

He leaned closer, brushing a gloved hand across the pubic hair, inspecting the skin underneath for any sign of rash, scratching, inflammation, or the scars such things can leave behind. Laurie would have been deeply offended to know he was looking for signs of veneral diseases, but she would have been even more deeply shocked to know how often he found them. Obstetricians and gynecologists hear more than their share of denials, rebuttals, and outright lies, and early in their careers they learn never to take anything as gospel unless they see it themselves.

Gently, with one finger, he opened the labia, noting the healthy pink color inside. He located the clitoris, which was normal, inspected the tip of the uretha just below it for signs of infection and, finding none, moved on to the introitus, the opening of the vagina itself.

Testing the entranceway with a finger, he confirmed more of what Laurie had told him. Nulliparous: no previous deliveries. A baby's head leaves an unmistakable imprint of stretch marks and scar tissue when it passes the introitus. Crenshaw spoke quietly to the nurse, who went to a drawer, selected a speculum of appropriate size, took it to the sink, and ran warm water over it before handing it to him.

With the speculum in place, Crenshaw bent to examine the inside of the vagina. It was a glossy pink, lined with the sharp ridges that are characteristic of a normal healthy vagina. At the back, he could see the tiny, smooth knob of the cervix. It was a slightly darker pink than the rest of the vagina, another bit of data to bolster the diagnosis of pregnancy. In pregnancy, the blood vessels in the cervix expand, giving it a bluish cast.

But most of what Crenshaw could see was negative, and that was reassuring. There were no signs of any inflammation, no blood or pus around the cervix, no abnormal formations that would suggest cancer. There were no ridges on the cervix, and that was especially reassuring; such ridges are characteristically found in women whose mothers took the now-infamous drug DES to prevent spontaneous abortion. There was no vaginal infection. Those were so easy to spot that taking a culture was only for confirmation. A yeast infection would have left a residue that strongly resembled fine-curd cottage cheese. Trichomonas, the other common vaginal infection, would be gray-green and frothy.

The nurse handed Crenshaw a long wooden stick with an eccentric double knob at one end. Crenshaw carefully guided the knobbed end through the speculum and up against the cervix.

With an expert twirl of his fingers he rotated the double knob so that the inside portion turned a full circle at the center of the cervix, while the other knob rubbed along the organ's entire circumference. Withdrawing the stick, he rubbed the knobs across a glass slide and handed both items to the nurse. The nurse then handed him a long stick with a moistened cotton swab on the end. Crenshaw pressed the swab gently against the center of the cervix until the head of the swab moved slightly into it, then twirled the swab and withdrew it. The sample went onto a second slide, completing the Pap smear.

The procedure, a routine in every gynecological examination, is especially important during pregnancy. It is rare for a pregnancy to be complicated by the sudden onset of cervical cancer, but it happens often enough to be worth checking for. Later, a laboratory technician would examine the slides, looking for the deformed cells characteristic of cancer.

The Pap smear done, Crenshaw took one final glance through the speculum for reassurance, then closed it and removed it. He reached for a tube of sterile lubricant, smeared a dab of it on his gloved right hand, and slipped two fingers into the vagina, feeling for the cervix. In a normal, healthy woman who is not pregnant, the cervix will feel hard and gristly, like the tip of a nose. In pregnancy, the cervix becomes engorged with blood and begins to soften. This early in a pregnancy the softening was slight and subtle, but Crenshaw could, he thought, notice a difference. More data. More reassurance.

Then, as he pressed down on Laurie's abdomen with his free hand, he felt the cervix along its entire length. Another occasional complication of pregnancy is a condition known as incompetent cervix. An incompetent cervix dilates more easily than it should, and as the baby grows larger and gravity puts more pressure on the cervix, the cervix begins to give way. Often, in the second trimester, the woman spontaneously delivers. Such babies almost never survive.

This early in the pregnancy, Crenshaw would be unable to feel the funnel shape that is characteristic of an incompetent cervix, but he wanted to know as much about it as his fingers could tell him. Was it long or short, firm or soft? Did it appear to be in the proper location? Were there any bumps—potential tumors—along its length? There were none. It felt normal. More data. More things he could rule out.

Then his attention moved to the far end of the cervix, where it merges into the uterus. Again his hand pressed against Laurie's abdomen, his fingers reaching back and forth to try to feel the lower aspect of the uterus. He could not. Good. That, too, was normal. A normal nonpregnant uterus is roughly the consistency of a ripe tomato. In early pregnancy, blood flows to the lower uterus and makes it so soft that often the upper part of the uterus feels like a separate organ. Again his hand pressed against the abdomen. There it was, right where he expected. Fine. More data. More reassurance.

Now he began to press against different parts of Laurie's abdomen, trying to turn the uterus slightly, stretching out his fingers for more details. Were there any lumps that could be fibroid tumors or cysts on the outside of the uterus? There were none. Good. Rule that out, too.

"Tell me if anything hurts," Crenshaw reminded Laurie, as he began feeling around for her fallopian tubes. If he found one, it would be a very bad sign. If Laurie gasped with pain when he found it, that would be worse—a strong sign of tubal pregnancy or, worse, of ovarian cancer. But Laurie remained quiet and he found no sign of swollen fallopian tubes. As he probed with his fingers, he found both ovaries, right where they should be. One of them was somewhat enlarged, just as it should be in a newly pregnant woman. More data, still negative, still reassuring.

Finally, he directed his fingers to just beyond the far end of the cervix, testing the cul-de-sac between the cervix, the end of the vagina, and the uterus, named the Pouch of Douglas after the anatomist who first described it. Tumors might grow there, or cysts. Ovaries and tubes could deform and protrude into the space. It didn't happen often, but Crenshaw never failed to check.

Then, withdrawing his second finger from the vagina, he moved it slightly downward and slipped it into the rectum, while the index finger went back into the vagina. The rectovaginal exam is uncomfortable, and certainly ignoble, but it provides data that is especially useful when the patient is pregnant.

The second finger can reach higher and farther back into the pelvis through the rectum than it can through the vagina, and now Crenshaw felt around for the bony archway at the rear of the pelvis called the sacral promontory. With his thumb on the tip of the pubic bone and his finger brushing the sacral promontory, Crenshaw could make a remarkably accurate estimate of the size of the birth canal, something that would be important about eight month hence.

By moving his second finger from side to side, he could also feel the two rather sharp prominences, called spines, that flanked the sacral promontory and marked its widest dimension. By comparing height with width, he could judge the birth canal's shape, and the shape was almost as important as the size.

During labor, a full-term baby's head becomes elongated, almost cone-shaped, to allow it to fit more easily through the birth canal. In a normal, round birth canal, the mother's contractions will push the baby through the passageway headfirst, with the head bowed and occiput, the back of the head, coming out first. The baby emerges looking at the floor.

If the canal is anthropoid, a flat oval shape, the baby will often come out looking at the ceiling, which is not a problem for the baby, but it can damage the mother's upper vagina and uretha. If the canal is android, roughly heart-shaped, there may not be enough room for the baby's head at all. Women with small android birth canals once died slow, agonizing deaths, suffering increasingly painful contractions until finally the uterus itself burst and the women died in a river of blood. Nowadays such women have children by cesarean section, and an experienced obstetrician can often tell during the first examination whether the operation will be necessary.

As the information from Crenshaw's fingertips accumulated,

in his mind he formed a three-dimensional picture of a pelvis. This one was ideal: gynecoid in shape, and large enough to accommodate a normal-sized baby. Nothing that would warn of a difficult delivery. More reassurance.

That done, Crenshaw moved his fingers upward, taking further advantage of his increased reach to feel the far wall of the uterus, the part that is usually beyond the fingertips in a vaginal exam. It was smooth and firm and presented no cause for worry.

Finally, he brushed his two fingers against each other, inspecting the wall of tissue, called a septum, between vagina and rectum. Occasionally, rarely, a doctor will discover a rectal tumor that way, and if the diagnosis is early enough, he may save a life. Again, he found reassuringly negative data. He withdrew his fingers, pulled off the examining glove, and dropped it in the trashcan.

He pushed the stool back from the examining table and stood up. "Everything seems fine," he told Laurie as he walked back to the office. "Come next door when you get dressed, and we can talk." He closed the door, sat down at the desk, and reached for his Dictaphone with one hand as he lit a cigarette with the other.

[5]

The First Scare

IT IS UNUSUAL—rare, in fact, these days—for a physician to smoke. Carlyle Crenshaw acknowledges that, sometimes several times a day. He is the only member of the ob/gyn faculty who smokes, and his faculty members remind him of this with almost missionary zeal. It is his prerogative as department chairman to ignore all the good advice, but he has, in fact, tried to quit several times. It never works. The nicotine craving conjures up the old nightmare, every time, of the day he smoked his first cigarette.

When he was in college, Carlyle had bought a pipe and begun to smoke it. At first it was only for effect—he thought the pipe made him look older, more serious, wiser. It also gave him an advantage in any conversation: If he needed a pause to collect his thoughts, he only had to take the pipe out of his mouth, look at it, tamp the tobacco down with a thumb, strike a match with some ceremony, light the pipe with several deep puffs, then squint through the cloud of smoke and say, casually, "Now, what was the question?" It gave him something to do with his hands. Like many honor students, Carlyle was mildly compulsive; he liked to stay busy, he said. During the long, quiet hours when he studied, the pipe was in his mouth constantly. Often it was unlit, and even when it was lit he didn't inhale the smoke, but the pipe was a pleasant substitute for fidgeting, a sort of socially acceptable pacifier.

When he entered medical school at Duke, the pipe went with him. After he graduated and began his one-year internship, the pipe helped keep him awake during the long nights on the hospital floor. By the time he began his residency, it was an institution; wherever Carlyle went, the pipe jutted out of his mouth. In those days surgical masks were worn in the delivery room. Soon the nurses began to joke that they'd have to make Carlyle a special mask with a hole in it, so he could smoke his pipe in the delivery room.

One of Crenshaw's fellow first-year residents, Robert Jackson, kidded him unmercifully about the pipe. Crenshaw could add two or three useful hours to his day, Jackson would say, if he would quit fiddling with that silly goddam pipe all the time and smoke cigarettes instead. Once, he had gotten Crenshaw to take a puff from a cigarette, but after the rich taste of a pipe, the cigarette smoke tasted thin and flat, faintly unpleasant. He handed the cigarette back. "You didn't inhale," Jackson said accusingly. "You have to inhale cigarette smoke." Crenshaw grinned and began loading his pipe. Crenshaw and Jackson were often paired together on duty, and the good natured harassment went on during every smoke break. Jackson would offer Crenshaw a cigarette, Crenshaw would refuse and begin stoking up his pipe.

First-year residents traditionally work the labor and delivery suites. The job is mostly routine, mostly long, dull hours of waiting and watching, occasionally standing at the foot of the delivery-room table to catch babies at the end of normal, uncomplicated labors. First-year residents are not expected to handle the difficult cases; they are expected to notify their senior colleagues. If a mild complication develops during labor, the first-year man calls in a second- or third-year resident. If the problem is unusual or instructive, several other middle-level residents will hear of it. It must be severe before the chief resident is disturbed. The chief resident speaks directly to the attending, the faculty member with ultimate decision-making authority, and residents learn early not to waste the time of the chief or the attending. On the other hand, woe betide the resident who waits too long to notify the top brass. It is a delicate balance—one of the ways residents learn to make the fine judgments expected of senior physicians.

Nothing was at all unusual one particular morning when young Dr. Crenshaw arrived, promptly at 7:30, to attend morning rounds with the residents who'd worked the night before. There had been two uncomplicated deliveries during the night;

the mothers and infants were all doing well. Only one woman was still in labor; she'd come in two hours earlier and was progressing normally—rapidly, in fact, for a primigravida. All her signs were fine except her blood pressure, which was a tiny bit elevated: 130 over 90, instead of the usual 120 over 80. Not ominous, but worrisome, and worth watching. Crenshaw chewed on his pipe and watched. He made sure a nurse took the woman's blood pressure regularly, and it stayed rock steady at 130 over 90. He watched a while longer, then walked back to the nurses' station and lit his pipe.

The woman's labor progressed normally and rapidly, and after a comparatively short time, the nurses wheeled her down the hall to the delivery room. There the woman pushed and strained, but she seemed to be making little progress. Crenshaw was hardly surprised, since the woman was petite—she was nine months pregnant and weighed only one hundred pounds. Crenshaw could tell with his fingertips that the birth canal was wide enough for the baby's head, but only barely. The tiny woman pushed, pushed, pushed, and got nowhere. Perspiration rolled down her face; clearly, she was in great pain and her strength was ebbing. Something had to be done.

"Forceps," Crenshaw ordered. Working rapidly, he numbed the perineum with local anesthetic, then made an incision along one side of the bulging introitus to widen the opening. Carefully he maneuvered the forceps into position around the baby's cheekbones, and with a strong, steady tug brought the baby's head out the introitus. The woman gasped, then relaxed. The baby was a boy, and he yelled as soon as he could draw a lungful of air. A tough delivery, but not too tough. Perhaps he should have called in a higher-level resident, but there really hadn't been time and things had gone fine. Crenshaw quietly congratulated himself for being such a thoroughly competent first-year resident.

The mother's strength returned rapidly, and she complained, as most new mothers do, while Crenshaw stitched up the places where her perineum had torn. The stitches hurt, she complained, and besides, she was *hungry*. When could she get something to eat? Soon, Crenshaw said, soon. It wasn't exactly the truth, but not exactly a lie either. No food was allowed in the delivery room, and all new mothers were required to stay in the delivery room for an hour after giving birth so the residents could be sure they didn't bleed catastrophically and their blood pressure stayed normal.

That was a bit more of a worry with this patient since her blood pressure was slightly up. Her record said that her blood pressure was normally 110 over 70, a little low, so 130 over 90 was more remarkable for her than for most. Crenshaw had heard horror stories about preeclampsia that went undiagnosed, and he jolly well didn't want one of those while *he* was in charge. He double-checked the lab results he'd gotten earlier, but the two urine samples, collected at different times, showed no protein. That was reassuring because preeclamptic women nearly always had protein in their urine. And they often had pain in the upper right quadrant, the area just below the right breast. The pain was from swelling of the liver capsule, but patients described it as a stomachache. And preeclamptics usually became high-strung, nervous, irritable about everything. Indeed, that triad of symptoms, irritability, stomachache, and proteinuria, were a red flag that not even a first-year medical student should miss, much less a resident.

Crenshaw watched and waited. The woman described, in increasingly plaintive terms, how hungry she was, but there was no stomachache. They stalled her by returning her baby to her, fresh from his first bath, and she was allowed to nurse him while she was still on the delivery-room table. The nursing served a dual purpose. It took the mother's mind off lunch, and the act of nursing, the stimulation of her nipples, caused her uterus to contract more rapidly, making it less and less likely that she would develop postpartum bleeding.

At the end of an hour, the woman's blood pressure was still rock-steady, 130 over 90. Except for that, she was in perfect shape. "Give her sixty of phenobarb," he told the nurse, "and check her BP every four hours." Sixty milligrams of phenobarbital wasn't enough to put her to sleep, but it should lower her blood pressure. Crenshaw made sure a lunch tray would be delivered to the woman and sent her back to her six-bed ward room. Then he went to lunch himself, filling and lighting his pipe on the way.

When he came back, he stopped in the ward to check on his patient. She was fine, she said, but she was getting sick of listening to the patient in the next bed. The ward had privacy curtains, but they didn't reduce noise. The patient in the next bed was a seventeen-year-old girl who had, two days before, delivered a fine, healthy baby. The girl's mother had stayed with her almost constantly, and the fact that the girl wasn't married had been a point of serious discussion between daughter and mother. The girl was being discharged that afternoon, and the arguments had risen to hysteria; twice, the other women in the ward had had to call the nurses to quiet both the mother and the daughter. They'd been fighting all along, Crenshaw's patient told him, but today the young girl seemed incredibly ill-tempered. On his way out, Crenshaw made it a point to stop and chat with mother and daughter. The presence of an authority figure such as Dr. Crenshaw had a calming effect on both of them. Soon Crenshaw had them smiling; he promised to expedite the paperwork for them so that they could leave early.

Crenshaw was at the nursing station, on the phone, arguing with the admitting office when a nurse came racing down the hallway and skidded to a stop in front of Crenshaw. "Seizure," she panted, "we've got a seizure." Crenshaw dropped the telephone receiver next to his pipe on the desk and raced for the ward. The petite woman lay rigid on her bed, teeth clenched, eyes rolled back, quivering. A nurse already had a pressure cuff around the woman's arm. "One-sixty over one-ten," she reported.

Crenshaw stared aghast, betrayed by his textbooks. This was eclampsia. A fully eclamptic patient meant the resident *missed* the symptoms of preeclampsia, and in all of obstetrics there is no more unforgivable sin. This woman hadn't had any of the textbook symptoms of preeclampsia, but there'd be no explaining that to the chief resident.

"Mag sulfate," he snapped at a nurse. "Get me five hundred of mag sulfate solution, and a quarter of morphine." The nurse fled out the door, almost bumping into Jackson, who'd been working in an adjacent wing and had heard the fuss. They stood, one at each side of the bed, working frantically. The woman's pupils contracted rapidly when Crenshaw shined a light in her eyes, but her body remained rigid, and she made no response to their increasingly urgent exhortations.

The nurse returned with the prescribed medications, and very quickly they had the desired effect. The magnesium sulfate began to lower the woman's blood pressure, and the morphine relaxed her taut muscles. Crenshaw added a dose of barbiturate to prevent further seizures. Soon the woman blinked her eyes and stared at the doctors with a puzzled expression. Crenshaw let out a long breath.

It was then that he realized they had an audience. The mother and daughter from the adjacent bed had been timidly standing at a distance during the entire crisis. The daughter was dressed, her baby wrapped in a flannel blanket, ready to leave. Crenshaw walked over to them, apologized for the delay, and gave them directions to the admitting office. They thanked him politely and left.

A gaggle of residents began to arrive on the ward—word of a disaster spreads like wildfire through a hospital. Second-, third-, and fourth-year residents came running, and before long the chief resident himself appeared. The crisis was over and the chief listened attentively as Crenshaw self-consciously described the lack of symptoms that had preceded the seizure.

At the chief resident's suggestion, a nurse used a catheter to take a fresh urine sample from the woman. Sure enough, there still was no protein in the urine. The residents drew a blood sample and had it analyzed for uric acid, another sure sign. It was normal. The woman's blood pressure was back to 120 over 80 now, but with all the drugs she had in her blood, it had to go down. The chief resident agreed: a most unusual case.

They summoned a senior resident in neurology, who shined lights in the woman's eyes, tested her reflexes with a rubber hammer, and pricked her skin in several places with a safety pin. No, he finally announced, he saw no signs of epilepsy, or anything else that would explain a seizure. Sorry.

The committee of residents had adjourned to the nurses' station by then, leaving a nurse in the ward to check the patient's blood pressure every fifteen minutes. The chief resident was talking about another eclampsia case he'd seen, when a nurse at the desk inquired, "Who's on duty?" Crenshaw turned around, and the nurse handed him a telephone. It was the emergency-room resident. "We have a woman down here with seizures. Her mother says she was just discharged from OB. Can you come look at her?" The blood drained from Crenshaw's face. No. This could not be happening. Not twice in one afternoon. Not two eclamptics, two *undiagnosed* eclamptics, not, please, by all the gods of medicine, two of them happening to the same first-year resident in the same day!

Chagrin did not slow him down. "Robert," he called, and, with a brief explanation to the others, the two first-year men galloped down the stairway and raced to the emergency room. They arrived out of breath and stood panting while the ER resident described the girl's symptoms. Body rigid, teeth clenched, eyes open but unfocused—it was the same thing all over again.

Crenshaw went to the girl's bedside, where a nurse was checking her blood pressure again and again, looking puzzled. "I'm getting one-twenty over eighty," the nurse said. Crenshaw stared at the girl, who remained rigid on the bed. Then he saw her eyes blink. He spoke her name sharply.

The girl's body remained rigid, quivering, but her mouth moved. "What?" she said huskily, then clenched her teeth again.

Crenshaw felt a great weight vanish from him. He spoke to the girl again. "Why are you doing this?" he asked gently.

The girl relaxed, then burst into tears. "I don't want to go home with my mother," she sobbed. "All she does is yell at me."

Crenshaw stroked the girl's hand and sent a nurse to fetch a mild sedative for her. Then he conferred with Jackson and the ER resident, and the three of them went to the waiting room, where Crenshaw spoke to the girl's mother. "She appeared to have a seizure," Crenshaw said, dancing around the edges of the truth. "She's fine now. The best way to prevent this from happening again is to keep her very calm; don't do anything to upset her." The mother promised, and the three residents left solemnly.

Out of sight of the mother, Crenshaw collapsed against a wall and laughed quietly. Then he patted his pockets. Damn. Damn! His pipe was several hallways and several flights of stairs distant. And right now, more than anything in the world, he wanted . . .

"Jackson," Crenshaw said, "gimme a cigarette." He lit the short white cylinder and drew in a deep lungful of smoke, then another, then another. Later that day, he bought a pack of his own.

Two days later, the chief resident presented the cases of the surprise eclamptics—the real one and the fake one—at the department's grand rounds. Crenshaw didn't attend the presentation; he was delivering babies. Afterward, the chief sought out Crenshaw in the hallway and told him the department chairman had a message for him. Crenshaw raised an eyebrow.

"The message is this," said the chief. " 'You only get one. That's your quota. If you ever get another one, you can look for another job.' " Crenshaw stared thoughtfully at the chief resident's back as he walked away.

It is a matter of record that Carlyle Crenshaw never had another eclamptic. He has had near misses, and he has treated a great number of other people's eclamptics, but he has never had another of his own. But to this day, any hint of preeclampsia conjures up the scowling ghost of his old department chairman, and he watches those patients with extra vigilance. And he still smokes cigarettes.

He lit another one as he finished dictating his observations about Laura Edwards. Her blood pressure had been 130 over 90, that magic figure that had betrayed him once before. He had double-checked the nurse's reading, and it was correct.

Thirty years of experience had taught him that a great number of women have mildly elevated blood pressure during late-life pregnancies, and that very few of them develop problems. The best thing to do was to wait, and to monitor blood pressure closely. In most women, that slightly elevated blood pressure would drop during the second trimester, and when that happened, the chances of any complications would be slim. Not nonexistent, but slim.

Stubbing out the cigarette, Crenshaw reached for Laurie's folder and wrote, carefully, "Watch for hypertension."

[6]

Common Sense

WHEN Laurie walked back into the consulting room, Crenshaw was busy filling out what appeared to be another machine-scored form like the one she had already completed. She sat down in the chair opposite his desk and watched. Shortly he raised his head, looked at her over his glasses, and smiled. "I wish all my patients were as healthy as you," he said. "I can't find much to criticize. If it weren't for your blood pressure, which is a little bit high, I'd say you are in perfect health."

Laurie smiled at the compliment, but then the lawyer took over. "We were going to talk about risk," she said.

Crenshaw paused briefly. "The fact that you're—"he glanced at the chart "—thirty-eight years old does put you at risk. Now let me tell you what that means statistically."

He settled back in his chair and removed his glasses, the professor at a seminar. "The normal background risk of having a baby with any sort of birth defect at any age is between two and three percent and, remember, that's an average of all the worst cases with all the best cases. But let's say it's three percent.

"At thirty-eight—" he glanced at the chart again, did a quick mental calculation "—thirty-nine when you deliver, the risk of Down's syndrome is between six and ten per thousand, depending on who you listen to. The risk of having any other chromosomal abnormality is about twelve per thousand.

"That, in obstetrics, is considered high risk, and because of that I'm going to recommend that you come in for genetic counseling, and also that you have an amniocentesis to see if there are any anomalies.

"If we did find a serious genetic defect, you would have to decide whether you wanted to terminate the pregnancy or not.

Hopefully, that's a decision you'll never have to make, but it's something you ought to talk over with your husband. If you decide you would never have an abortion under any circumstances, then there's no reason to go through the amnio. We do have patients who want the test anyway, just so they'll know, but we recommend against that, because the procedure itself carries a slight risk."

He took a deep drag on the cigarette. "I want to be sure to keep this risk business in perspective. When we say high risk, we're talking about an average risk of about five percent. Turn that around, and you have a ninety-five percent chance of having a normal pregnancy and a healthy baby.

"If you were twenty-two, that would be ninety-seven or ninety-eight percent. That extra two or three percent of risk is what puts you in the high risk category.

"But those are averages. They don't take into account the overall health of the mother or the type of care she gets. I would never be foolish enough to promise you a perfect baby, but your odds are very good."

Laurie shifted in her chair and looked as though she was about to say something, but Crenshaw went on. "There are a number of things you can do to improve those odds, too. The most obvious one is diet. You'd be amazed at how many pregnancies I see that are high risk simply because the mother's malnourished. The best advice I can give you is to use good sense. Eat well-balanced meals: lean meat, fish, fowl, fresh vegetables, salads. Try to stay away from processed foods and sweets. It's a good idea to have a snack before you go to bed at night. Drink milk, lots of it, a quart a day."

He paused, wrote briefly on a prescription pad, tore off the sheet and handed it to Laurie. "This is for extra-strength multiple vitamins and an iron supplement. You'll need plenty of both."

"What about gaining weight?" Laurie asked.

"We're not fanatic about that either," Crenshaw replied. "For someone your size, we'd like to see you gain about three pounds a month, so that at term you weigh twenty-five to thirty pounds more than your prepregnant weight. There are some months when you'll gain more and some when you'll gain less, but an average of three pounds a month is about right.

"We have the same philosophy about exercise. And I can tell from looking at you that you exercise regularly."

"I play tennis," Laurie said. "I was going to ask you about that."

"There's no reason to stop, as long as you play in a sane fashion, and that's true for any sort of exercise," he replied. "Exercise doesn't increase risk as long as you don't go to extremes. Anything you already do, that you're already in shape for, you can continue to do. But try to avoid getting too winded. You might want to play doubles, so you don't work quite so hard—" Laurie winced mentally "—but there's no reason to stop as long as it's comfortable for you to play.

"In fact," he said, "women who exercise regularly have significantly shorter labors and easier deliveries than women who don't. Just be sensible about it."

Crenshaw paused and Laurie seized her chance. "We talked about the risks for the baby a minute ago. Aren't there other risks? What about my blood pressure?"

"There are indeed," Crenshaw replied. "Principally there are two. One is diabetes, the other is high blood pressure. Those are things that often occur later in life, but sometimes they also occur during pregnancy and go away after delivery. When they do arise, they're a risk to both the mother and the baby.

"Your blood pressure is a trifle high. It's one-thirty over ninety, which ordinarily would not be alarming. I imagine that if you cut down on your salt consumption, your blood pressure will drop back to normal.

"That small elevation should not be a problem for a pregnant woman either, and in the vast majority of cases it isn't. But in a business where five percent is high risk, we take things like that very seriously.

"One of the reasons we'll want you to come in for regular checkups is so we can watch your blood pressure. The closer to term you get, the more often we'll check you. We'll want you to bring in a urine specimen every time you come for a checkup. That's very important. We send that to the lab, and it can tell us all sorts of things. If we find protein in it, we'll worry about your blood pressure. If we find sugar in it, we'll worry about diabetes. If we don't see either, we'll still worry a little, but not as much.

"And if we do see any signs of either diabetes or high blood pressure, that's not a disaster by itself; we have a lot of experience dealing with both those conditions, and there are a number of things we can do to control them.

"At your age, there's also a very slight risk of premature labor, and if you're prone to urinary tract infections, that increases the risk a little more.

"That's not anything to worry about this early, but it brings up a point I really like to stress, and that is participation." Crenshaw leaned forward, resting his arms on the desk. "You have to be a participant in managing this pregnancy. You are the best monitor we've got. You're going to be the first one to realize it if something's not quite right, and it's your responsibility to call and report it right away.

"This," he said, writing on a slip of paper, "is the phone number of our group's answering service. They always know which one of us is on call. You call them, they'll beep us, and we'll phone you right back.

"And if, God forbid, that doesn't work, this second number is the direct line to our delivery suite here. There are nurses and physicians there twenty-four hours a day. Any time you think something might be wrong, you should call one of us or call the delivery room. We may tell you not to worry, or tell you to come in first thing in the morning, or tell you to come in right away. The important thing is that if you're worried, you should always phone."

"What sort of thing would I be likely to call about?" Laurie asked.

"I don't want to put limitations on what you should call about. If you're worried, call. Now, if you call to tell us your ankles are swollen, or your breasts are tender, we'll probably tell you not to worry about it.

"The things you ought to be especially sensitive about are spotting, or any leakage of any kind, particularly early in the pregnancy. Any sharp abdominal pain. Later in the pregnancy, any tightening of the abdomen that lasts for very long, or occurs more than twice. That might be premature labor. We can almost always stop premature labor if we can get to you early enough. That's one area where your awareness is critical.

"In general, any sudden change. If your stomach hurts, call. If you get spots in front of your eyes, call. If your mood suddenly changes, if you get extremely nervous and agitated, call. Anything that seems important to you probably *is* important, and you ought to call us. If you're in a car wreck, for example, we'll want to monitor the baby's heartbeat to make sure he's okay.

"And that brings up another important point: seat belts. There's a lot of misinformation about seat belts and whether you should wear them. You should. You should wear the belt as low on your hips as you can, and wear your shoulder harness normally, so the strap's not directly over your middle. If you do have an accident you'll do better, and so will the baby, if you have your seat belt on."

Crenshaw shifted back in his chair, lit another cigarette. "And that's about it, except for the standard warning about intercourse. I like to recommend that couples stop having intercourse about four to six weeks before the due date. That's a very conservative attitude on my part, and there are some very good doctors, including some in this department, who say it's fine right up until you go into labor. But there are studies that suggest a connection between intercourse, orgasm, and premature labor. I'd as soon not take the chance.

"I also have to mention, uh, oral sex." For the first time in the interview, Crenshaw looked slightly uncomfortable. "This offends some people, but you need to know that it's extremely dangerous to let anyone blow in your vagina when you're pregnant. It can cause an air embolism, and you can die within a couple minutes.

"And that's about it," he said. "I don't see any reason to worry about your pregnancy at this point. We'll want to see you again in four weeks, which will give you time to think about whether you want the genetic counseling and amniocentesis."

"When would you do the amniocentesis?" Laurie asked.

"Generally during the sixteenth week," Crenshaw replied. "We don't like to do them any later than that."

Laurie thought a moment. "I suppose," she said slowly, "that if I'm going to be my own monitor, as you said, I should read up on the subject. Can you recommend something?"

"There are a number of books," Crenshaw replied. "Most book stores have a good selection. I'd say just pick out one that interests you."

"I was thinking more along the lines of a textbook," Laurie said.

Crenshaw winced. "I wouldn't recommend a textbook, and I hope you won't go out and buy one. It'll make you worry about things you shouldn't worry about. I treat a lot of doctors and doctors' wives, and they are the worst patients, because they always go back and dig up their textbooks. It just causes trouble."

Laurie started to argue, then thought better of it. "Okay," she said, noncommittally. "That's all the questions I have. Are we done?"

"Yep," Crenshaw said. He stood up, walked to the door, and opened it for Laurie. "I'll see you in a month."

Crenshaw followed Laurie out into the lobby, picked up the next chart, called out the name, and escorted the next patient into his office. Laurie walked up to the nurse's desk. "How much do I owe you?" she asked.

"Nothing right now," the nurse replied. "You get a bill for the whole thing after you have your baby."

Laurie whistled appreciatively. It would probably be quite a bill, considering. Thank heaven for insurance, she thought.

"How about exactly four weeks from today?" the nurse asked, reaching for an appointment card. Laurie nodded. The nurse wrote the date and time on the card, handed it to Laurie. "Want me to stamp your ticket?" she asked.

"Ticket?" Laurie replied.

"For the parking garage. If we stamp it you only pay half price."

Laurie remembered the parking meter, and looked at her watch. "I parked on the street," she said. "But thanks, I'll remember that next time." Laurie left hurriedly, found the elevators, waited a seemingly interminable time, and finally got to the first floor. She walked briskly, almost at a trot, through the lobby, ran a short way down the sidewalk until she could see her car, then stopped, cursing. Under the windshield wiper was a parking ticket.

[7]

Dr. David Nagey

THE NEXT DAY, Laurie bought a text-book on obstetrics and a medical dictionary. Within a week, she bitterly regretted it. She'd attacked the book, *Williams Obstetrics,* 16th Edition, with the same ferocious concentration she'd brought to bear on her law books. The first night, she'd read about the normal symptoms of pregnancy. When she read that oil glands around the nipples become distended in pregnancy, she stopped, went into the bathroom, and checked. Sure enough, there were tiny lumps in her areolae. Impressed, she returned to the book, read that many women experienced nausea, headache, and backache during pregnancy. She congratulated herself on having avoided all those symptoms.

The next day she had all three. She didn't quite throw up, the headache wasn't quite bad enough to keep her home from work, and the backache wasn't either. She'd also read that aspirin was discouraged during early pregnancy, so she toughed it out and by afternoon she felt fine. She and Bill even played tennis that night, but for the first time in a long while, Bill won easily.

Laurie was not the sort to believe in superstitions, or in hypochondria, or even the power of suggestion, so when she and Bill got home from the tennis courts, she resumed her reading. It was slow going, because the language was unfamiliar. She kept the medical dictionary open on her lap and rested the heavy textbook on the arm of her chair.

The chapter on female reproductive anatomy had been illuminating. She had never paid terribly close attention to her own, and she became engrossed in a detailed sketch of the external female genitalia. She concentrated, memorizing the official names and locations of things she had known only by touch. She was tempted to get a mirror and make comparisons, but the idea seemed somehow unacademic, so she continued reading instead.

She was equally fascinated by the drawings of the internal reproductive organs. The cervix surprised her; it was larger than she'd imagined, and barrel-shaped, with thick fleshy walls that extended upward from the upper edge of the vagina. The uterus was smaller than she'd expected, really just an extension of the cervix, it seemed from the diagram. What distinguished the two, she read, was that the walls of the uterus were composed primarily of muscle, while the walls of the cervix were of connective tissue, tougher and less elastic than muscle.

She was surprised again when she realized that the ovaries were attached to the outside of the uterus, with the fallopian tubes curling around the ovaries before turning inward. For reasons she couldn't recall she'd had the impression that the ovaries sat higher in the abdomen, connected to the uterus only by the fallopian tubes, the way the kidneys connect to the bladder.

Now, for the first time, the pelvic exam made more sense to her. From the drawing she could see that it was possible to feel the front part of the uterus through the vagina, while the back portion was more easily accessible through the rectum. She promised herself she'd remember that, next time.

The next night she read that she would be likely to develop varicose veins, hemorrhoids, and stretch marks. She might have heartburn, excessive fatigue, and "leukorrhea," an increased vaginal discharge of mucous material. She did feel tired, she thought, but her only other symptom was occasional heartburn, and she'd had that for years.

The following night, she began reading about the things that could go wrong. She could have an ectopic pregnancy. The fertilized ovum could have stayed in the ovary, or in the fallopian tube, or could have migrated through the uterus and down into the cervix. She was reassured to read that severe pain was a symptom of all those disorders. She felt fine, actually.

She read about *placenta previa*, where the placenta formed across the bottom of the uterus and bled during labor, and *abrup-*

tio placenta, in which the placenta separated prematurely from the uterine walls. Both were accompanied by severe bleeding and led occasionally to the death of infant, mother, or both. She read about spontaneous abortion. Half the spontaneous abortions could not be traced to a specific cause, the book said. They just happened. She skipped over the part about elective abortions; she didn't want to know just yet.

Then she read about hypertension and diabetes, about cervical cancer during pregnancy, about anemia, thyroid diseases, collagen diseases, viral and bacterial infections, endocrine disorders, and diseases of the nervous system during pregnancy. She'd never dreamed there were so many things that could go wrong! She read about dystocia, abnormal labor. It could be caused by a misshapen pelvis, by a defective uterus or cervix, by a baby in the wrong position, by . . . by almost anything. An entire smorgasbord of things could go wrong during labor.

And afterward, as well. She might bleed excessively after delivery, or the placenta might not come out as it should. The uterus could turn itself inside out and protrude from the vagina. She could get an alarming array of infections, some of which were treated by immediate hysterectomy . . . .

By the time four weeks had passed, Laurie had read most of the textbook and was desperate to be examined. Remembering Crenshaw's reaction, she was equally determined not to give away the fact that she'd gotten a textbook. She might have tried simply to brazen it out with rapid-fire cross examination, but she knew she probably wouldn't have understood all the medical jargon and it would have been bad form to carry the dictionary with her.

The morning of the exam, she headed straight for the bathroom as soon as she awoke, and found the jar she'd so meticulously washed the night before. The jar had once contained olives, and it had a tight-fitting lid with a rubber seal. Both Crenshaw and the nurse had told her to be sure and save her first urine of the day, because it always gave the best test results. This time, when it didn't matter, she didn't spill a drop. She twisted the cap into place, set the jar on the back of the toilet, and stepped into the shower.

There was a parking space on the street again, but Laurie ignored it and parked in the underground garage across from the hospital. She got to the private offices nearly ten minutes early, handed over her urine specimen, sat down, and discovered to her utter amazement that the magazines in the office were current. There was one other woman in the waiting room, sitting at a right angle to Laurie, reading *People* magazine. The woman was pregnant, attractive, and about Laurie's age. She wore a loose-fitting maternity dress, but from the size of the bulge beneath it, Laurie guessed that the woman was about halfway through her pregnancy. And, Laurie thought as she looked closer, the woman might even be a little older than she was.

The woman felt Laurie's gaze, looked up and smiled. "Are you one of Dr. Nagey's patients?" she asked.

"I think I'm Dr. Crenshaw's patient, actually," Laurie said, "but I think that means I see all of them."

"It does." The woman's eyes darted to Laurie's waist, then back to her face. "How many weeks?" she asked.

Laurie thought for a moment. "Ten," she said finally. "About ten."

"Have you been depressed?" the woman asked. "I always get real depressed about then."

"I worry a lot," Laurie confessed, "but I wouldn't call it depression. This isn't your first?"

"No, it's my fourth—or my third; I never know which way to count. I've had four pregnancies and one of them didn't work out."

"Oh, I'm sorry," Laurie said.

"Don't be," the woman answered. "It was for the best. We did the amniocentesis," she said, pronouncing the word casually, "and it showed we had a bad baby. So we had to . . . to stop the pregnancy. That was six months ago. I got pregnant again right away."

"God, you must be terrified this time. This is only my first, and I'm scared to death something will go wrong."

"How old are you?" the woman asked bluntly.

"Almost thirty-nine," Laurie answered, a trifle sheepishly.

The woman chuckled. "Count your blessings. I'm forty-four." Seeing Laurie's expression, the woman went on, "I've got two daughters, eight and eleven. My husband and I decided we'd like to try for a boy."

"But the risk . . . " Laurie paused.

"One in ten," the woman said matter-of-factly. "And if this one doesn't work out, we'll give up. But we wanted to try."

"I see," Laurie temporized. She was vaguely uncomfortable with the sudden intimacy of the conversation, but at the same time she recognized the potential gold mine of information. Abruptly, she shifted the subject. "What's the amniocentesis like?" she asked.

"Unpleasant," the woman said. "Not much fun, but not nearly as bad as you think it's going to be. It doesn't hurt, or not much anyway. But I guarantee you, you'll worry yourself sick over it. I just had my second one, and I think I dreaded it even more than the first. Take my advice and look at the ceiling the whole time."

Laurie suppressed a shudder. "Thanks," she said.

"The advantage," the woman went on, "is that you get to see your baby on the ultrasound monitor. That part is great."

"How long do you wait before you find out . . ." Laurie left the rest of the question unspoken.

"I'll know in another week. It takes two or three weeks usually. You get the results quicker if they're bad, because they want to give you as much time as they can to, to . . . make up your mind."

"Oh," Laurie said. "Yeah, That must be—"

"Sad," the woman finished the sentence for Laurie. "It was very sad. The baby would've had Down's syndrome." The woman's voice grew flat, uninflected. "We had talked about it ahead of time, and we knew what we had to do, but it was still tough. It was probably the toughest thing I ever had to do in my life. I didn't feel angry, or guilty, or anything like that; I was just sad. Trish stayed with me the whole time while I had the abortion; that helped a lot.''

"Trish?" Laurie asked.

"Oh, you haven't met Trish yet? That's who I'm waiting for now. Trish is the . . . '' the woman looked puzzled. "You know, I don't know what her title is. Trish teaches childbirth classes, and she does other things, too, and she works with high-risk patients. She . . . '' the woman paused again, thinking. "She's sort of an ombudsman, a patient advocate. If you don't understand something, or you don't like something, you can talk to Trish, and it's not like talking to a doctor; it's like talking to an old friend.''

"Trish is a doctor?" Laurie asked.

"No, no. Trish is a nurse. It wouldn't work if she was a doctor.''

Laurie started to ask what wouldn't work, but right then she heard someone say "Mrs. Edwards?" She looked up, startled, to see a young, blond, heavyset man in a white coat standing in front of her with a chart in his hand. She stood up, and the man held out his hand. "I'm David Nagey," he said. "Dr. Crenshaw's at a conference this week, so I'm seeing his patients. Come in." Laurie stood, nodded a quick farewell to the other woman, and followed Nagey through the door.

In the consulting room, Nagey opened her chart, leafed through several pages, then ran a finger down one. "Your lab studies from last time look great," he said without preamble. "The urinalysis was good, the blood studies were all normal, and so was the Pap smear. Your blood pressure was a little higher than we'd like, but not alarmingly high. We'll want to keep an eye on that, but it's not something you ought to spend any time worrying about." He looked up. "How do you feel?"

"Fine," Laurie answered automatically. "Apprehensive, in spite of all the advice," she added.

"You wouldn't be normal if you weren't," Nagey said with a

grin. "Everybody worries. It goes with the territory. Can I answer any questions for you?"

"I've been hearing a lot of horror stories about things that can go wrong in a pregnancy, particularly when you're my age." Nagey nodded politely, waited for her to continue. She thought a moment. "Oh, what the hell. I bought a textbook." Nagey winced, then smiled but still said nothing. Laurie continued. "It was a mistake. I know it was a mistake, Dr. Crenshaw warned me it'd be a mistake, he was right, I admit it, and now I know about all these horrible things. Torn placentas. Myomas. Infections. I get frustrated sitting around waiting for those things to happen. I feel like I ought to be doing something."

"You are," Nagey said. "You're eating right, exercising, drinking milk, not smoking, not drinking, and taking vitamins. That's actually quite a lot.

"But let me go down the checklist and see if we can help put your mind at ease. Have you had any vaginal bleeding?"

"No," Laurie replied.

"Any fluid at all from your vagina?"

"No."

"Any puffiness or swelling in your face or fingers?"

"No."

"How about headaches?"

"One or two. They went away."

"Dizziness? Blurred vision? Ringing in the ears?"

"No."

"Pain? Any abdominal pain at all?"

"No."

"Nausea? Persistent vomiting?"

"A little nausea. No vomiting."

"Chills? Fever? Anything like that?"

"No."

"Trouble urinating? Urinating too frequently?"

"Neither."

Nagey leaned back in his chair. "You certainly don't sound like someone who has cause to worry," he said. "But let's go next door and let me listen to your tummy, just to be sure."

Laurie had been prepared, indeed almost eager, for another pelvic exam, and was mildly surprised when Nagey said there was no need for one. Instead, he took her blood pressure and then directed her to loosen her skirt and blouse and lie down on the examining table. Nagey reached into a cupboard and took out a green plastic electronic device with stethoscope-like earpieces attached to it.

He explained that it was a Doppler monitor, and that it operated by sending an ultrasonic signal into her abdomen and measuring the bounce-back. The explanation was more technical than Laurie could follow, so she laid there, mystified, and made polite noises.

Nagey squeezed some clear gel out of a tube and rubbed it on her abdomen. It was so cold it raised goose bumps. Then he pressed the device firmly against her abdomen and began sliding it around, tilting it one way, then another. Finally, he held one position for a long time, and consulted his wristwatch. Then, holding the device in place against her stomach, he removed the earpiece and offered it to Laurie.

"Would you like to listen?" he asked.

"What is it?"

"It's your baby's heartbeat."

Laurie put the earpiece on and heard a rapid, high-pitched, liquid sound, the unmistakable ta-dump, ta-dump, ta-dump of a heartbeat. She felt a sudden surge of emotion; her lungs congested and she felt her eyes begin to mist over. Reluctantly, she handed the earpiece back to Nagey and said, huskily, "Thank you."

[8]

Trish Payne

DR. NAGEY'S OWN EYES were moist as he put away the Doppler stethoscope. A decade of experience had not diminished his capacity for empathy, nor did he want it to. In medical school and during his residency, both his professors and his peers had warned him to keep plenty of emotional distance between himself and his patients, lest he begin to feel their feelings and share their sorrows. His replies were more or less polite, depending on the status of the person giving the advice, but his opinion of the advice was unchanging: It was horse hockey. Why would you go into obstetrics if not to share in the thousand little thrills your patients felt? You were bound to share the occasional tragedy, perhaps spill a few tears, but not often. Obstetrics, even high-risk obstetrics, was a business of happy outcomes. If it weren't, Dave Nagey would have been an engineer.

He had started out to be an engineer. He had a remarkable aptitude for mathematics; so remarkable that by age fifteen he had run out of math courses to take in high school. His solution was simple enough: He dropped out of high school and enrolled in college. He got an engineering degree from Purdue University when he was eighteen. Then a summer job in a medical lab convinced him he should be a bioengineer, so he enrolled at Duke University Medical School, just to learn the language. He quickly came to hate all the rote memorization and all the hard work, but he decided to hang on until he could rotate through a few clinical departments and get some hands-on experience.

His first rotation, by chance, was obstetrics, and suddenly he was fascinated. By tradition, an OB rotation begins with a visit to the delivery room, and the erstwhile bioengineer stood enraptured as he watched, for the first time, a child being born. Now, *there* was a job of bioengineering, he thought admiringly. He contrived to spend as much time as he could in the delivery room after that, to admire and study this impressive phenomenon. He quickly learned the essential facts, details, and procedures of delivery and discussed each case in detail with the delivery-room resident. Eventually, the moment came when the resident, at that last crucial moment before the baby's head was about to emerge, stepped away from the end of the table and said to Dave, "You do it."

Behind his surgical mask, Nagey opened his mouth to protest, then caught himself. This is the only way you learn it, he reminded himself, so he fought back the stage fright, forced his mind onto the details of labor and delivery, pulled on a pair of sterile gloves, and stepped into position.

The birth was, as the resident had known it would be, uncomplicated. The mother, a large, somber woman, had borne several other children successfully; her labor had been brief and efficient. Now she endured the pain of delivery stoically, a great funereal scowl on her face.

Soon, Nagey stood crouched at the end of the table holding a squalling baby, while a nurse clamped and cut the umbilical cord. He held the baby up and watched the woman's frown melt into a smile that widened and widened until it seemed to light up the entire room. He was hooked. He knew it even before he realized that the event had taken place on his own twentieth birthday.

He struggled to hang onto an engineering career, and in fact he earned a Ph.D. in biomedical engineering from Duke the year before he received his M.D. But obstetrics had replaced engineering as his first love and, as soon as he finished medical school, he enrolled in Duke's medical-resident training program. He hated the first part of his residency for the same reasons that he'd hated the first part of medical school, and once he even went looking for engineering jobs, but his professors urged him to stay on. One of those professors was Duke's director of high-risk obstetrics, Dr. Carlyle Crenshaw.

Dr. Crenshaw saw in the young resident a resource that obstetrics could ill afford to lose; there were precious few obstetric scientists who truly understood mathematics. Crenshaw enlisted Nagey in several research projects, and Nagey worked out mathematical formulas to explain the biological and medical phenomena involved. It was almost as much fun as delivering babies. Nagey finished his residency, won a two-year fellowship at Duke, and became an assistant professor at age twenty-nine. After Dr. Crenshaw left Duke to move to the University of Maryland, he phoned Dr. Nagey one day and invited him to switch jobs. Nagey thought about it. Would the department buy him a computer so he could continue his mathematical modeling projects? he asked. Sure, Crenshaw replied.

The computer sits, largely unused, on a desk in Dr. Nagey's office. Between supervising residents, teaching, lecturing, keeping an eye on all the construction projects the department has under way, and seeing patients and delivering an occasional baby, Dr. Nagey has little time left for the computer. He has a grant to start a pilot project for computerizing birth records throughout the state of Maryland, but his role is that of supervisor rather than inventor. More than anything, he wants to devise a computer program that will record data, minute by minute, or even second by second, from the delivery suites themselves, and store that data so that, in a few months or a few years, he can begin to say mathematically and medically sound things about the childbirth process. For someone whose twin loves are bioengineering and obstetrics, this is the stuff dreams are made of.

His problem is, he enjoys it all. The teaching is fun, and so was helping to design the new labor-and-delivery suites and overseeing their construction. He works on his mathematical models in his spare time, like some people work crossword puzzles, and working with the residents is a pleasure. All those things are fun and sometimes he wishes he could spend more time at them. But if he did, there would be less time to spend with patients like Laura Edwards. There would be fewer occasions when, as just now, he could use the Doppler stethoscope to introduce a mother to her new baby, fewer occasions when he could see the sudden flush of emotion and the tears of joy that are so contagious. For him, this is the real payoff.

Nagey carefully wiped the gel off the Doppler stethoscope before he replaced it in its case, then put the case back in the cabinet. He turned back to Laurie and saw from her expression that she was still working to digest the experience. He hated to intrude, but there were more patients to see, more work to do, and there was never enough time. He went to the door that led to the consulting room, opened it, then turned to Laurie. "Come next door when you get dressed," he said. "I need to talk to you a little more."

Laurie's thoughts were in turmoil as she refastened her skirt and blouse. She was at once thrilled and frightened, and her thoughts were solemn and profound. Before, she had merely been pregnant, Laurie thought. Now, she was *with child*. The thing in her belly, still so small she could hardly see a bulge, was not an embryo, not a fetus; it was a baby. Her baby.

She finished straightening her clothes, and returned to the consulting office. The room seemed softer than she remembered, and Nagey, five years younger than Laurie, seemed somehow older, fatherly and wise. Much later, when she recalled the moment, she would observe that the experience had temporarily switched off her intellect and had placed her emotions in control. At the time, she only knew that she felt slightly puzzled, very euphoric, and more of a woman than she could ever remember.

"I want to reassure you," he began, "that everything seems completely normal. I'd like to tell you not to worry, but I know it wouldn't do any good. It's natural to worry, and my philosophy is that it's even good to worry a little; it shows you care about your baby.

"However," he said, "I really think you ought to hide that textbook somewhere for a few months. You'll worry about all the wrong things if you keep reading the textbook."

"What do you mean?" she asked.

"Most of the things in the textbook are very rare, and you'll never get any of them, no matter how much you think you will. If you're going to worry, why not put it to good use? Worry about things that are realistic risks."

"Such as?"

"Such as car wrecks. Do you wear a seat belt when you drive?"

"I do now. Dr. Crenshaw mentioned that."

"I'm sure he did. So will I. So will everybody here. The risk of you losing your baby in a car wreck is greater than all the medical risks of pregnancy put together. Did you know that?"

Laurie stared. "I hadn't heard it put quite that way, no."

"It's true." Nagey reached into a desk drawer, brought out a pamphlet and handed it to Laurie. She looked at it. The pamphlet's title was *Should I Wear A Seat Belt While I'm Pregnant?* Laurie figured she knew the answer by now.

"Okay," she said. "I'm convinced."

Nagey grinned. "You'll hear it again, I guarantee. This is something we're fanatic about. Keep that pamphlet; it tells you how to wear the belt."

The euphoria of a few moments before was fading quickly now, and the lawyer part of Laurie's mind was taking over again, steering the conversation back to other questions.

"Surely there are a few things besides car wrecks that I can worry about," she said, arching an eyebrow.

"Worry is not the right word, really. There are things you ought to be aware of and watch out for. If you want to worry, worry about missing them.

"First, some things related to your blood pressure. It's not high enough to worry about, but it makes us cautious. You ought to watch out for several telltale symptoms. For example, any sudden weight gain. If you suddenly start to get puffy, call us; we'll probably want to check you right away. The same goes for headaches, dizziness, spots in front of your eyes, ringing in your ears, that sort of thing.

"We also want to be on the lookout for any symptoms that might suggest diabetes. Excessive thirst and excessive urination are two things to watch for.

"We check the urine specimens you bring in for other signs of those two problems, too, so it's very important that you not forget to bring them. Later on in the pregnancy, we'll probably do a quick diabetic screening test, just to ease everyone's mind.

"Then, about halfway through the pregnancy, we'll start watching for any sign of premature labor, but that's still a few months away. Those three things are your principal concerns and the things you should watch for the most closely."

Nagey shifted in his chair. "The one other area we need to talk about," he said carefully, "is the genetic risk. It's not terribly high, but it is measurable, and for that reason we suggest you have genetic counseling and amniocentesis. I'm sure Dr. Crenshaw brought it up. Have you thought about it?"

Laurie suddenly felt defensive. All the talk of risks hadn't really bothered her until just then, but the mention of something that might threaten her baby stirred up a great primitive hostility. She felt an impulse to shout "No!" but she suppressed it, and the lawyer part of her mind quickly began to chide her for being irrational. She stared at Nagey for a long moment, then dropped her eyes before she finally answered. "I've thought a lot about it," she said, "and I've talked it over with my husband. The idea terrifies me, but I know it's the only sensible thing to do."

"It won't be half as bad as you expect it to be," Nagey said, as he pushed back his chair and stood up. "That's everything I need to tell you this time," he said. "Let me take you out and introduce you to Trish Payne. Have you met Trish?"

"No, but I've heard about her," Laurie said. "What exactly does Trish do?"

"I call her our high-risk coordinator," Nagey replied, "but she does a little bit of everything." He ushered Laurie out of the consulting room, down the green-carpeted hallway to an open door. Inside, in a tiny, cluttered office, sat a woman in a jade green scrub suit, bent over, writing in a notebook on her lap. Nagey tapped on the open door, and the woman looked up, broke into a cherubic smile, and said hello.

"Trish, this is Laurie," Nagey said, simply, then turned to Laurie. "We'll see you in another four weeks. Be sure to see the nurses out front before you leave." With a wave of his hand, Nagey turned back toward the examining rooms.

Trish gestured toward an empty chair in the room. "This is the best office they'll give me," she complained with a chuckle. "Make yourself at home. Dr. Bennett told me she talked to you."

"Dr. Bennett?" Laurie asked, puzzled.

"Norma Bennett. She said she met you in the waiting room."

"Oh. I didn't know she was a doctor."

"She's a dentist. So's her husband. They're a wonderful couple. They're going to come here for childbirth classes, if . . . " Trish let the sentence trail off.

"I know," Laurie said. "She told me. She told me quite a lot, actually, in a short time."

"She does that. That's how she deals with it. She's going nuts right now, but you'd never guess it. She's so calm and matter-of-fact about everything."

"How soon will she know?"

"Soon. A week, probably. Chances are, she'd have heard something already if it was bad news, but that's not always true. You never really know until you get that call from the lab. And they don't call until they're sure. I almost offered to call them and see what I could find out, but I didn't, thank goodness. It's always a temptation, but imagine if I told her everything was fine, and then it turned out everything wasn't fine. She'd be devastated, and so would I."

"Sounds like the worst part of an amniocentesis is the waiting," Laurie observed.

"It is. You can't help but think about it. The only reward, really, is that the overwhelming majority of tests give good results, and getting that good news is such a high—it's almost as big a high as actually having the baby. Have you made up your mind whether you want it?"

"I don't *want* it," Laurie said, "but I'm going to have it done. At my age, I'd be foolish not to."

Trish made a face. "Poo," she said. "If you tell yourself you're too old too often, you'll start to believe it. Let's see, you're . . . "

"Thirty-eight," Laurie said. "Almost thirty-nine."

"That's not old. That's the prime of life." Trish smiled again. "Do you know why thirty-five is the magic number where high risk supposedly begins?"

Laurie thought about it. "No," she said carefully. "I've always heard thirty-five, and never really stopped to question it. If I had to guess, I'd say that thirty-five is where the risk starts to become measurable."

"That's a good guess, but it's not quite right," Trish said. "If you study large enough groups of women, you can measure risk at any age. We know that under eighteen is a very high risk group, and we know that from about eighteen to about thirty-five is the lowest-risk group. But there is that background risk, and if you look at it very closely, you can see that it starts going up a long time before thirty-five?"

"Okay," Laurie said. "So why thirty-five?"

"Let me back into that. You know what amniocentesis is for?"

"Sure. To detect Down's syndrome."

"Well, genetic or chromosomal defects. Down's is the most common, and it's one of the ones for which probability increases with age. Anyway, you also know that there's a small risk involved in the amniocentesis?"

"I assume so, but I don't know what it is."

"It's about three per thousand, or one in three hundred."

"One in three hundred what?" Laurie asked. "What am I risking?"

"That within a week of the amnio you'll have a miscarriage. A certain number of women miscarry, and a certain number of them miscarry at between sixteen and seventeen weeks. Women who've had amniocentesis increase that risk by about one in three hundred." Trish leaned forward. "Now. Guess what age you have to be before the risk of genetic defects exceeds one in three hundred."

Laurie smiled. "I would bet heavily that it's thirty-five."

"Right." Trish beamed, then sobered. "One of the real ironies is that more Down's babies are being born to women *under* thirty-five now than to women *over* thirty-five. You can't screen the women under thirty-five because you can't justify the risk.''

''You mean I can't have amniocentesis unless I'm over thirty-five?''

''No, anybody can have it, but we advise against it. Some people insist on having it anyway. They say it's available, why not use it? Some of them—a lot of them, in fact—are husbands pushing their wives into having it because they want to be sure they have a perfect baby.''

Trish shuffled through the stack of papers that was still on her lap. ''Speaking of perfection,'' she said, ''are you going to come to childbirth classes and learn how to have the perfect labor and delivery?''

Laurie looked up, saw Trish's smile, and smiled back. ''How could I say no to a deal like that?'' she replied. ''When do we start?''

''Oh, not for a long time. Thirty weeks or so. Ideally, you'll walk out of your last class and go right into labor.''

''I've heard you're good, but I bet you're not *that* good,'' Laurie grinned. ''Do I get my money back if I don't have a perfect delivery?''

Trish laughed. ''Absolutely not. All the classes really do is prepare you for childbirth. The idea is that there should be no surprises left by the time you go into labor. You experience a lot of things in labor that you'll never experience any other time in your life, and they can be frightening if you don't know what they are. And if you're frightened, you can't enjoy the experience.''

''Enjoy?'' Laurie cocked an eyebrow.

''Okay, appreciate may be a better word. Childbirth can be a very negative experience, or a very positive one. You go to classes to learn how to make it a positive experience.''

''I'm sold,'' Laurie said. ''Where do I enlist?''

''You just did. I'll let you know a few weeks before the classes start. I'll be talking to you before then, anyway. Has anybody told you what I do?''

"No. They've tried. It sounds like you do a little of everything."

"I do. But my real purpose in working with the high-risk patients is to make sure nothing gets overlooked. Even in the very best places things can fall through the cracks. I'm sort of a safety net for that. I'm . . . well, available. Accessible. If you have a question, or you're worried about something and you don't want to call the docs, you can call me. If they do something that you don't understand, or that you don't like, I can tell you what's going on, or I can go yell at them for it. If they don't explain things to your satisfaction, I can try. I guess I'm sort of the person in charge of loose ends."

"You'd better be careful," Laurie observed, "or you'll turn the hospital into a pleasant place."

Trish giggled. "Heaven forbid," she said. "We have enough trouble getting people to go home as it is." She shuffled her stack of papers again. "Back to business—have you scheduled your genetic counseling yet?"

"No. How do I do that?"

Trish wrote a name and number on a slip of paper, handed it to Laurie. "This is the genetic counselor. You and your husband need to meet with her ahead of time so she can explain all the procedures, and the risks, and get all the paperwork ready. You'll probably meet with her a week or two before you come in for the amnio."

[9]

A Case of Eclampsia

LAURIE drove back to her office and tried to put in an afternoon's work, but her mind swirled with thoughts of high blood pressure, amniocentesis, her forbidden textbook, and, most of all, Dr. Norma Bennett. She even consulted the phone book, found an office number for "Bennett Norma R DDS," and jotted it down, but she didn't call; she couldn't decide how she would begin the conversation. Finally, she was able to distract herself with a long, complicated contract that she had been asked to review. More and more of her time was being spent providing second opinions for the other partners. Her phenomenal memory and her eye for detail had become one of the firm's principal assets.

That night, Laurie handed her textbook over to Bill. "Put this somewhere," she instructed him, "and don't tell me where." Bill looked puzzled. "Don't ask," she said. "You don't want to know. Just do it." Without a word, Bill disappeared into the basement, and returned a few minutes later without the book.

There were negotiations that night. As their lives had settled into workaday routines, Bill had resumed his role as chief cook, and the meals he prepared were uniformly delicious. Many of them, however, contained varying amounts of salt. Laurie, acting on Crenshaw's advice, had asked Bill to reduce the amount of salt. Now, after learning that her blood pressure was still high, she asked Bill to leave out the salt completely. He started to protest but she cut him off. "You can still salt your own food after it's cooked," she reminded him.

Bill obliged, and that night he fed Laurie a meal of baked chicken, steamed broccoli, and boiled potatoes, with no salt in any of them. The food looked wonderful but tasted unbelievably bland. Laurie dutifully ate it all, and after dinner she just as dutifully fought back the cigarette craving which, somehow, had been made worse by the bland meal. She fidgeted awhile, tried to read and couldn't. She wanted to read the textbook, she wanted a cigarette, she wanted salt, she wanted a snifter of brandy—she wanted everything that was forbidden. Finally, with a long sigh, she hoisted herself out of her chair, walked to the kitchen, and poured herself a tall glass of milk.

Over the next four weeks, Laurie tried hard to grow accustomed to salt-free food. She visited a bookstore and bought *Craig Claiborne's Gourmet Diet* and Michel Guerard's *Cuisine Minceur*. Bill, who read cookbooks the way Laurie read history books, was appropriately grateful, and immediately set about experimenting with various combinations of spices designed to fool the low-sodium palate. He concocted a salt-free sweet mustard that, when mixed with oil and vinegar, made a remarkably good salad dressing. He made a salt-free spaghetti sauce that reeked of garlic, and a chili that was so hot Laurie never noticed the missing salt.

Several times, Laurie picked up the phone to call Norma Bennett, but each time she hung up without dialing. She should have called the same day, she told herself. What would she do now if she called up and found out that Dr. Bennett had gotten bad news and had had another abortion?

Finally, she called Trish. They chatted about various subjects while Laurie worked around to the question she wanted to ask. Finally, she began hesitantly, "I've been wondering about Dr. Bennett. Have you heard anything about her?"

"Only that the results were good, the baby's healthy and she's on top of the world," Trish said airly. "Other than that, no. Why?"

"That's what I wanted to know. I've thought about calling her several times, just to talk, but I didn't want to phone to talk about having babies if she had just . . . " Laurie couldn't bring herself to pronounce the words; she let the sentence trail off.

"I see what you mean," Trish answered. "I'm sure she'd

love to talk to you. She couldn't be any happier. It's a boy, you know.''

"How does she know?"

"The amnio. They can look at the chromosomes and tell. They'll tell you what it is, if you want to know. A lot of women don't want to know. I wouldn't. I'd rather be surprised."

Laurie thanked Trish for her help and hung up. Then she sat at her desk for a long time, thinking. Finally, she picked up the phone again and dialed Dr. Norma Bennett's office.

Her fourteen-week exam was performed by Dr. Crenshaw, and it, like the ten-week exam, consisted of the urine specimen, the blood-pressure check, and the Doppler stethoscope exam. Laurie listened to the fetal heartbeat again, but this time the thrill was not the same, and she noted that the sound most nearly resembled the squishing noise some people make when they rinse their mouths.

As before, the nurse took Laurie's blood pressure, and then Crenshaw took it himself. He seemed pleased. "Your blood pressure's down a little this time," he announced. "It's one twenty-five over eighty-five. That's a really good sign."

"I've stopped eating salt," Laurie responded. "Nothing tastes right without it, but it looks like it's working."

"Maybe," Crenshaw said thoughtfully. "Sometimes it will drop even if you don't do anything, but either way it's a very good sign. When your pressure drops during the middle trimester, it means your chances of having blood-pressure problems during the rest of your pregnancy are a lot less."

Later, in the consulting room, Crenshaw brought it up again. "Your blood pressure may well go back up during the third trimester," he warned Laurie. "We'll want to watch you very closely then, and if it does go up and it stays up after the baby's born, you probably ought to start taking medication for it, but not until after the pregnancy's over. Until then we want to avoid giving you any sort of medication, because we don't really know which ones are safe during pregnancy.

"Watching your salt intake will help, both now and later, but you don't have to be fanatic about it. You can still eat bacon once in a while; just don't overdo it.''

When the interview was over, Crenshaw ushered Laurie out and said goodbye, then returned to his desk and carefully noted his findings in her medical record. The dip in blood pressure was very good news, but he would be wary nevertheless. Toxemia was a rare complication and its symptoms are usually easy to recognize, but, as he knew all too well, there are exceptions. Some cases, like the one that happened during his residency, were simply bad luck. There were some that were inexcusable.

Like Patricia Williams. It always made Crenshaw's gastric juices curdle to think about Patricia Williams. She was young, poor, black, single, and pregnant for the first time. She was nineteen years old and eager to have the baby. The baby's father was a mechanic, and was equally thrilled by the pregnancy. As soon as he could find steady work and find a place for them to live, he said, he wanted to get married.

Late one hot summer afternoon, Patricia Williams showed up at the emergency room of her community hospital complaining of severe headache and stomach pains. She was seen by a young surgeon, not long out of his residency, whose specialty was hernias and bowel resections, and who resented his periodic ER duty. He examined Patricia, noted on the chart that her blood pressure was 130 over 100 and that she seemed distraught. He would be distraught, too, if he lived in an unairconditioned public housing project on a day like this, he thought. He prescribed antacids for the woman's gastritis and sent her home.

Four hours later Patricia came back to the hospital, even more agitated. The antacids hadn't worked, she complained. She still had the headache and the pain on her right side was worse, not better. What she needed, the surgeon figured, was a tranquilizer, but he remembered enough from his obstetrics course to know that you don't prescribe tranquilizers for pregnant women. So he gave her more antacids and sent her home again.

The third time Patricia came to the hospital it was in an ambulance, unconscious, convulsing. The surgeon took one look at her and told the ambulance to take her to the University of Maryland Hospital, fast.

On the way there, the woman stopped breathing. The ambulance attendant gave her mouth-to-mouth resuscitation until they got to University's emergency room, where an anesthesiologist forced an airway tube down her windpipe and then trotted alongside the gurney, squeezing air into her lungs with a black bag, as the ambulance crew took her straight to the obstetric floor.

It happened to be Dr. Crenshaw's night on duty, and he and two residents were waiting when the gurney arrived. Within seconds they had given her morphine and magnesium sulfate and, as soon as the ambulance crew lifted the woman onto a delivery-room bed, they attached fetal-monitor probes to her abdomen. A strip of graph paper began to emerge from the monitor, a tracing of black ink across its face. Crenshaw and the residents studied the readouts of the monitor and examined the strip of paper. To be sure, they listened for a long time with Doppler stethoscopes. There was no fetal heartbeat. The baby was dead.

"Stat section?" a resident inquired. This was by the book. Immediate—"stat," in medical jargon—cesarean section was the proper last-ditch treatment for severe eclampsia. But Crenshaw was examining the woman's head, holding back first one eyelid and then the other, shining a light across them.

"I don't think it matters," he said quietly. The pupils were wide, unseeing. Normally the bright light would have shrunk them to pinpoints. They didn't move. It was the grimmest of all neurological signs. The woman was brain dead. A neurologist confirmed Crenshaw's suspicion. The woman had had a massive stroke. She was undoubtedly brain dead. To satisfy legal requirements, the woman was moved to the intensive care unit, where neurology residents preformed two EEGs eight hours apart and confirmed the absence of all brain function. Then the respirator was disconnected and the body sent to the morgue.

The memory was enough to raise Crenshaw's own blood pressure. He never spoke to the emergency-room physician who missed such obvious signs of preeclampsia, but after looking over the hospital's records, he spoke at length with that physician's superiors. The conversation was cordial enough, but the message was clear. It was the same message Carlyle Crenshaw had received secondhand, from his department chairman so many years ago: You only get one. That's your quota, and now you've used it up. If it ever happens again, heaven help you.

[10]
Genetic Counseling

THE GENETIC counseling session required advance preparation. Laurie phoned Ann Jewell, the counselor, to schedule an appointment and got into a three-way negotiation over calendars when Jewell politely insisted that Bill attend the session. The very next day she received a letter from Jewell, encouraging her and Bill to contact all their blood relatives on both sides of the family to see if there were any cases of birth defects, mental retardation, or early pregnancy terminations.

Laurie was an only child, but her mother had come from a family of five girls, and her father had a brother and a sister. Both Bill's parents had come from medium-size families, and Bill had two brothers. Over the next few nights, they conducted a family reunion, piecemeal, over the telephone. Each phone call lasted longer than the previous one, as they chatted and passed along news of other relatives. One of Bill's uncles lived in Alaska, nobody knew where, and one of Laurie's aunts had died in an auto accident. Those were the only relatives they missed. There was one relative they later wished they'd missed: Laurie's Aunt Cynthia. Aunt Cindy lived in Pennsylvania, and she and her husband, a police captain, were active in several political groups associated with the far right. When Laurie mentioned genetic counseling, Aunt Cindy's voice grew sharp.

"Genetic what?" she demanded.

"Genetic counseling," Laurie repeated. She began to explain that they were trying to put together a family history so the geneticists could determine the chances of her baby having any birth defects, but Aunt Cindy cut her short.

"I won't tell you anything. There's nothing to tell, but if there was, I wouldn't tell you. You know what this is all about, don't you?"

There was no mistaking Aunt Cindy's hostility. Laurie tried to retreat. "Aunt Cindy, I'm . . . "

"Abortion," Aunt Cindy said, her voice almost a growl. "Abortion, that's what it's all about. Murder. You want an excuse to murder your unborn child."

There was no retreat. Instead, Laurie used her best crisp lawyer's voice and parried, "That's not what it's about, Aunt Cindy; I think you misunderstood me. We both want this baby very much. We hope we won't ever have to make that sort of decision at all."

"There is no decision," Aunt Cindy said, her voice rising. "There is no choice. Choice is a word murderers hide behind. Do you want to choose to murder your unborn child?"

"Look, Aunt Cindy," Laurie said firmly, "this is not what I called to talk about. I'd better go now. It was nice to hear your voice again. 'Bye now."

"You contemplate murder," the voice was even higher now, almost a shriek. "My niece, my sister's child, is a murderer!"

"Good-bye, Aunt Cindy," Laurie said firmly, and dropped the receiver back in its cradle. She brushed a hand across her forehead and realized she was sweating. She sank back into her armchair, looked at Bill, and signed. "I would give almost anything for a cigarette right now," she said.

Three weeks later, she and Bill parked in the university garage, consulted a map, then walked down Baltimore Street past the hospital building to a hulking red-brick tower called the Frank G. Bressler Research Building. They rode an elevator to the tenth floor and threaded their way down a narrow hallway littered with laboratory equipment to a door with signs on it that said 019 and DIVISION OF HUMAN GENETICS.

A slender, dark-haired woman wearing the standard badge of authority, a white lab coat, answered the door. She was obviously expecting them. "I'm Ann Jewell," she said, shaking hands with each of them. She ushered them into a medium-sized room that had been made cramped by dividing it up into two office cubicles and a small waiting area, complete with a small table containing several back issues of *National Geographic*.

The waiting area, it turned out, was also the genetic counseling area. Ann disappeared into one of the cubicles for a moment and returned carrying a printed form and the large medical textbook she used in place of a clipboard. She sat down next to Laurie and Bill and got right to work.

She began with the standard questions, starting with correct spelling of names and ending with medical insurance. The whole procedure was quite expensive, Ann explained, usually about nine hundred fifty dollars including all the lab work. Laurie winced, but Bill didn't. He'd checked just that morning, he said, and learned that their medical insurance would pay the entire amount.

"God, what do poor people do?" Laurie wondered aloud.

"We have a special fund for that," Ann replied distractedly, still writing on the form. "The problem isn't poor people, it's working people who have no insurance." She looked up. "Ethically, we can't deny the procedure to anyone who needs it, so sometimes we have to give cut-rate deals." She glanced back at the form. "Do you know if Dr. Crenshaw referred you for any reason besides age?" she asked.

"Not that he mentioned," Laurie answered.

"Good." Ann then asked what was becoming a standard series of questions about Laurie's health—was there any spotting, any puffiness, frequent urination, abdominal pain, persistent headaches, spots in front of the eyes, blurred vision, any of the traditional danger signs in pregnancy. There were none.

"Did you ever use any sort of contraception?" Ann asked.

"I used to use a diaphragm," Laurie replied.

"Were you using it when you got pregnant?"

"No, not for a year or more."

"Good." There were studies, Ann said, that showed a higher rate of spontaneous abortion in women who got pregnant while using a diaphragm with spermicides. That was one more potential risk they could rule out.

"How about drugs, medicines?" Ann asked. "Do you take anything?"

"Not even aspirin."

"Good. Don't. There's no such thing as a 'safe' drug when you're pregnant. The same goes for any 'recreational' drugs. They increase the risk enormously. In fact, if you were ever a heavy LSD user, there's some additional risk even now." Ann paused, looked up from her form.

Laurie smiled. "No problems there, either," she said. "I've never used it."

"I wish I had more patients like you," Ann said. "Now, tell me about your family."

The pedigree took some time to construct. In addition to wanting to know about birth defects and miscarriages, Ann was interested in the general health of their relatives. Two grandparents still survived, both in their eighties now; of the others, one had died of cancer, three of heart disease. Two had been killed in a car wreck.

"Two grandparents and one aunt," Laurie mused. "Does that put me at risk?"

"Everybody's at risk for that," Ann replied. "Has anybody told you about seat belts?"

"Many times," Laurie said.

The discussion turned back to relatives. Ann wanted to know about Bill's parents, all their siblings, and all their siblings' children. That took some time. Bill recited brief genealogies for five aunts and four uncles, and two dozen or more cousins. It was a remarkable feat of memory. Out of all those, none had any birth defect that he knew of, and none was retarded. A couple of them were pretty dumb, though, he added with deadpan seriousness.

Of Laurie's three living aunts, the youngest had miscarried twice, but then had produced two healthy children. Aunt Cindy, Laurie had learned from her mother and the two other aunts, had three apparently normal children. The eldest aunt was now rumored to have breast cancer, but no one in the family would talk about it. Her father and mother were both alive and healthy.

Ann turned a page on the form, made a few notations, then looked up again. "That's a very good family history. There's nothing that would indicate any unusual risk.

"But that doesn't mean there's no risk," she went on. "At age thirty-nine there's a one-in-eighty chance of the child having some chromosomal abnormality. Half of that risk, or one in one-sixty, is for Down's syndrome. You know what Down's syndrome is?"

Laurie and Bill nodded.

"I should add that the effects of Down's syndrome range from mild to severe, with most cases in the moderate area. There's always some retardation, and many Down's-syndrome children have problems with their internal organs that require surgical correction. On the other hand, many of them can lead useful lives."

Ann brought out a chart, with tiny photographs of banded, wormlike things pasted onto it in pairs. "This is what the inside of a cell looks like. Inside each and every cell, your cells, my cells, your husband's cells, there are these chromosomes. There are forty-six of them, twenty-three pairs.

"In Down's syndrome," she said pointing, "there's an extra chromosome on the twenty-first pair. Down's syndrome is also known as Trisomy-21.

"Half your genetic risk is for Down's syndrome. Most of the other half is for trisomy of two other pairs, thirteen and eighteen. Those are generally worse than Down's syndrome. They almost always involve severe retardation, and physical defects as well.

"Now, besides those age-related risks, you have the normal background risk of birth defects at any age, and that includes the risk of neural-tube defects like hydrocephalus and spina bifida. That's why we recommend the amniocentesis. Combined with the ultrasound exam, it is an extremely accurate procedure for diagnosing these things.

"Chances are, of course, that we won't diagnose anything. One of the reasons I like this job is because most of the time I give good news."

Ann leaned forward slightly. "But I won't tiptoe around the fact that sometimes I have bad news. Not often, but sometimes I do. Have you thought about what you'd want to do if we found some serious problem?"

Laurie looked at Bill, and he looked back. "We think," Bill said slowly, "that to continue such a pregnancy would be a cruelty, to us and to the baby." Laurie nodded assent.

Everyone was quiet for a long moment. Ann made another note on her form, then looked up, brightly. "But before you get depressed, remember it's a decision you most likely won't ever have to make. Usually I only give good news."

"Hear, hear," Bill said softly.

Ann put the chromosome charts aside. "I also want to tell you about the procedure itself so you'll know what to expect. Do you know anything about amniocentesis?"

"More than I'd like," Laurie answered wryly. "This is probably a silly question, but how big a needle do you use?"

"It's not a silly question at all," Ann replied. "The first question most people ask me is 'How much will it hurt?' The answer is that what hurts most is the local anesthetic, which stings for a second when it goes in. The procedure itself is uncomfortable, but people don't describe it as painful. The actual needle is about four inches long, and about as big around—" she glanced around, looking for something to compare, finally lifted the pencil she was holding "—the needle's about half the diameter of the lead in this pencil. It's a twenty-gauge needle, if that tells you anything."

"It tells me all I need to know," Laurie answered. "Excuse me for being paranoid."

"Not at all; that's a normal, healthy reaction. Pregnant women are very protective of their bodies, and especially their abdomens, and for very good reason. It is perfectly natural for you to worry about being stuck with a needle. In fact, if you *weren't* worried, then *we'd* be worried, because you'd be signaling us that you weren't particularly concerned about your baby."

"I'm glad I'm normal," Laurie replied halfheartedly. Ann began describing the ultrasound exam, and Laurie continued to nod as though paying attention, but a milky film had descended over her consciousness. It was a fresh shock each time she realized that she was behaving just like every other normal healthy pregnant woman. To a lawyer, such transparent behavior is a fatal weakness, like erratic swimming in a nest of sharks. Laurie prided herself on her mental self-discipline, and the realization of another lapse made her angry at herself. She'd been behaving as if she were inventing motherhood; as if she were the first person who ever had a baby at age thirty-nine; as if the earth would wobble in its orbit if anything went wrong!

". . . like an X ray," Ann was saying. "You can see the baby moving, see the baby's heart, take pictures of it . . . "

Laurie's anger against herself was subsiding almost as rapidly as it had arisen, but as it did, she made vow after solemn vow to herself to hang onto a rational perspective, to avoid taking herself so seriously.

" . . . the local anesthetic is what everybody says is the most painful part of the procedure because it pinches and burns, about like a bee sting . . . "

Abruptly, Laurie concentrated on Ann Jewell. This was important. Ann was talking about the needle now.

" . . . wash off your abdomen with antiseptics, and use sterile drapes and gloves, because we don't want to take any chance of an infection . . . "

She would watch the whole thing, Laurie decided. She wouldn't close her eyes or turn her head away. She'd pay attention when it happened and the terror would go away. Now, *that* was rational.

" . . . you know about the needle. You feel pressure when it's going in, and a lot of patients sort of"—Ann drew in a quick breath—"gasp like that when the needle finally goes in and the pressure's relieved. Then we generally draw off about thirty cc's of fluid, and that's it . . . "

It didn't sound all that bad. She'd definitely watch. It would be illuminating. Not the sort of thing to panic about.

" . . . some of the fluid gets sent off to be analyzed for alpha fetoprotein, which can warn us about the neural-tube defects like spina bifida. We do get false positives, which is why we never make a diagnosis unless we can confirm it with the ultrasound exam. We usually get the alpha fetoprotein results first, in a week or ten days, and we call you as soon as we do . . . "

She'd never have gotten so far in the legal business if she hadn't been able to handle stress. Anxiety was just another form of stress. No problem. No debate.

" . . . spin the rest of the fluid in a centrifuge, which moves the cells to the bottom. We put the cells into four separate flasks, and put the flasks in two separate incubators, just to be safe. It takes about three weeks for the cells to grow, and then a few days to harvest and analyze them. If the first sample has anything unusual we stop everything and immediately check the other three, so we can notify you as quickly as possible. That's why I tell people the longer they have to wait for results, the better the results are going to be . . . "

She'd been spending entirely too much time worrying and not enough time doing important things like staying in shape. Worrying was probably bad for the baby, too.

" . . . encourage husbands to be present for the procedure, or if you can't be there, then some support person to be in the room with us . . . "

No need to drag Bill along for the procedure. It had been enough trouble just getting him free for this, and now he knew everything she did. Anyway, all the important decisions were already made.

"I'll make it a point to be there," Bill said.

Laurie looked at him, smiled distractedly. She felt numb, drugged. More than anything, she wanted to fall asleep.

Ann was talking again. "One of the things we can tell from examining the chromosomes is what sex the baby is going to be. Are you going to want to know right away, or would you rather let it be a surprise?"

Laurie saw Bill open his mouth to speak, and a sudden surge of adrenalin wrenched her out of her reverie. This was something she'd thought about and decided on.

"Surprise us," she said.

[11]

Amniocentesis

WITH ONLY RARE EXCEPTIONS, Wednesday is amniocentesis day at the University of Maryland, because that is the day when the ultrasound suite is reserved for the obstetrics department.

Ultrasound imaging, or sonography, is the least precise way to look at the developing fetus. It is also the safest. Even at sixteen weeks, when the pregnancy is nearly half over, obstetricians are extremely reluctant to expose a fetus to X rays, particularly in the amounts necessary for a CAT scan. In the future, perhaps nuclear magnetic resonance imaging, which uses magnetism instead of X rays, will replace the ultrasound scanner. But for now an entire technology, and indeed an entire craft, has grown around the imprecise art of sonography.

The machine itself is analogous to a high-frequency sonar transponder, which sends out sound waves and measures what bounces back. In the human body the junction of dissimilar tissues creates echoes, and the pulses from those echoes feed into a high-speed computer, which displays them on a video screen as images. Like ordinary X rays, the pictures appear blurry and indistinct, and the expert interpretation of sonographs has become an informal subspecialty of radiology. The skillful manipulation of the machinery has become a new medical-technological skill. Ultrasound technicians are not paid as much as radiologists, but they are well paid indeed, and they bustle from cubicle to cubicle, wearing white lab coats and no-nonsense expressions. At one hundred dollars, an ultrasound scan is one of the most reasonably priced diagnostic examinations available, which probably accounts for the department's brisk business.

Laurie and Bill had to ask directions to get to the second-floor ultrasound lab. There was no waiting room. Instead the hallway was lined with more of the airport-style chairs that seemed to be everywhere, and today the chairs were crowded. There were two other pregnant women besides Laurie, both accompanied by men. In addition there were two men and a woman in the standard hospital-issue pajamas and robes, and one very old woman who dozed in a wheelchair that had an IV bottle hanging from a pole attached to the back of the chair. There was one empty chair; Bill insisted that Laurie sit in it and she willingly complied. Her middle had begun to swell noticeably, and she had found that the added weight threw her slightly off balance and caused her to stand differently, which in turn made her feet hurt more readily. She sank into the chair with a sigh, and Bill took up station beside her.

After a few minutes, Ann Jewell walked out of the lab area, spotted Laurie and Bill, and beckoned to them. The schedule, she informed them, was no more fouled up than usual. Dr. Pupkin, who would be doing the amniocentesis, was delivering a baby at the moment, but had promised that he would arrive within the next half hour or so. Laurie, Ann suggested, should get ready for her ultrasound scan now, so she'd be ready as soon as the doctor arrived.

Getting ready for the ultrasound exam, it developed, meant being assigned to an empty dressing room—there was a row of them at one end of the suite, like in a department store—where Laurie was instructed to take off all her clothes and put on one of the ridiculous little open-at-the-back smocks that hospitals everywhere prefer. These particular gowns were of thin flower-print cotton. The room was, like all hospital facilities, a trifle too cold for a person wrapped only in a thin cotton smock, and Laurie sat on a wooden chair in the dressing room and shivered.

After a mercifully short wait, Ann reappeared and led Laurie across the suite to a curtained-off cubicle that contained an examining table, a large machine on a stainless-steel cart, a wooden chair, two stainless-steel instrument tables, and a bearded ultrasound technician. Ann helped Laurie onto the bed, then adjusted a white sheet over her legs, pulling it low over her hips until it just covered her pubis. The ultrasound technician stepped forward, and Ann left to fetch Bill.

With a minimum of conversation, the technician smeared ice-cold jelly across Laurie's abdomen, flipped a switch on the ultrasound machine, and picked up a device that looked like the "hotcomb" variety of electric hair dryer. It was connected to the monitoring equipment by a long cord. The machine made a faint high-pitched whine. Ann returned with Bill just in time to dim the lights. Then the technician pressed the transponder against Laurie's abdomen and got to work.

The screen on the ultrasound device resembled a small black-and-white television screen, but this one had a gridwork of lines painted across it. At the edges of the screen the lines terminated in painted numbers. The images behind the gridwork were narrower at the top and wider at the bottom, as if generated by some mysterious electronic windshield wiper.

The first few images that flashed on the screen were blurry and confused, as the technician moved the transponder steadily back and forth across Laurie's abdomen, tilting the device first one way, then another, sweeping it back and forth along its own axis.

Except for the whine of the ultrasound machine, the room was breathlessly quiet. The soft glow of the screen provided an eerie illumination for the little knot of people clustered around it. Laurie, the patient, was all but invisible. The white sheet had slipped a little, exposing a corner of pubic hair, but not even Laurie noticed. The ultrasound machine was positioned so she could see it too, and her attention, like everyone else's was locked on the screen. She forgot the cold, forgot the ignominy of her circumstances, almost forgot to breathe.

The images moved and swirled on the screen, but now and then a familiar shape appeared. Once, it seemed to form the profile of a baby curled up in classic fetal position, but the image faded almost as soon as it appeared. Finally, the technician picked a spot, held the transponder very still, and pushed a button. The image froze on the screen; there was a clunk and whoosh and the picture was recorded on film. He moved the transponder again, held it still.

When the next image appeared, Ann leaned forward and pointed to a spot on the screen. "That's the fetal heart," she said. Laurie and Bill stared. Sure enough, there was motion on the screen. It looked like a fish's mouth rapidly opening and closing.

"Looks normal," the technician commented. "You can see the ventricles." He moved the transponder a fraction, and the fish's mouth was bisected by a vertical line, showing the separation between the left and right chambers of the baby's heart. He pressed the button and the image froze.

The technician recorded several more seemingly meaningless images before they got to the fetal head. Then he held the transponder still, froze the picture in place, and measured the skull width by counting the number of painted calibration lines from one side of the image to the other. Ann jotted the number down, consulted a chart on the wall. "Seventeen weeks," she said. "That's just about right."

Laurie and Bill were both disappointed when the lights came back on. The technician disappeared and Laurie readjusted the bedsheet, while Ann located a box of tissues and helped Laurie wipe most of the gel off her abdomen. Then Ann excused herself and told them both to wait while she checked on Dr. Pupkin. Bill helped Laurie finish wiping off the gel, and when they were finished, he put a hand on her middle. "I'm glad I came with you," he said quietly.

"You're not here to have a good time, you're here to hold my hand," Laurie answered with mock severity. "The real show is going to be when I see that needle and panic, and you have to chase me down the hall in this silly goddam gown."

"Better you than me, sport," Bill grinned. "I'll hold you down while they torture you."

Ann reappeared and escorted them out past several other curtained-off cubicles to a long, narrow room with a smaller ultrasound machine and a bed at the far end. Ann helped Laurie onto the bed. Bill, at Ann's suggestion, stood at the end of the bed by Laurie's head. Laurie folded the pillow on the bed to prop her head up higher, then laid very still and breathed deeply. She was terrified, much more than she'd ever admit, but grimly determined to see it through.

Amniocentesis, in modern obstetric history, is not a new concept. Physicians and scientists have long been fascinated by the clear, slightly yellow liquid that surrounds the developing fetus. Often, when the protective membranes ruptured at birth, doctors would catch samples of the fluid and analyze it.

Early on, they learned that during the first months of pregnancy the fluid seemed to originate in the amnion, the inner membrane that surrounds the fetus, and so the fluid came to be called amniotic fluid. In its initial stages, the fluid's chemical content was remarkably similar to the blood plasma of the mother. Later in pregnancy, the fluid became rich in nitrogen-containing compounds such as urea. The baby, it turned out, swallowed amniotic fluid and excreted it as urine. The thought, while not aesthetically pleasing, was not terribly disturbing, either. Urine is sterile, and clearly it didn't seem to hurt either the baby or the mother.

Scientists who examined the amniotic fluid under microscopes often found individual living cells, called fetal fibroblasts, which suggested that the infants inhaled the amniotic fluid as well. The discovery was academically interesting, but of little practical value. Perhaps, if there had been enough of the cells, it would have been possible to examine their genetic structure and predict genetic defects in unborn children, but there were too few cells. Cells could be grown in laboratory cultures, of course, but that required expensive and difficult techniques, and while doing so would have been an academic triumph, nothing would have been gained. In practical terms, predicting genetic defects would have been an exercise in futility. Abortion was illegal. If a child had a genetic defect, it would be duly noted at birth. But archiac laws could not completely stall the advance of obstetric science and technology, and when, in 1973, the Supreme Court issued its landmark ruling legalizing abortion, the genetic diagnostic amniocentesis suddenly became a meaningful procedure.

Scientists already knew they could concentrate the fetal fibroblast cells by spinning the amniotic fluid in a centrifuge. They knew they could grow the cells in flasks of nutrient solution inside special incubators and in about two weeks have enough cells to examine. They knew that to screen for genetic defects, they needed only to wash the cells in chemicals that would explode the DNA strand into its component chromosome pairs. Each of the individual chromosomes had its own characteristic shape and could be easily identified by using a high-power microscope. To screen for Down's syndrome, for example, it was necessary only to look for the presence of an extra twenty-first chromosome. The ability to predict the existence of Down's syndrome made amniocentesis an attractive technique for obstetricians and an urgent necessity for parents who could ill afford the financial or emotional expense of rearing a defective child.

Statistically, the procedure itself carried some risk. Mothers who had an amniocentesis experienced spontaneous abortions at a slightly higher rate than those who did not. The difference was about one in three hundred. For Laurie, the risk of having a baby with a genetic defect was one in eighty. That made the risk acceptable. The odds were further shifted in Laurie's favor by the fact that her amniocentesis would be done at the University of Maryland Hospital, by Dr. Marcos Pupkin. As with other areas of medicine, the extent of the doctor's experience makes a vast difference in the outcome. Dr. Pupkin had been performing the procedure for more than ten years. He knew what to look for, how hard to try, when to quit. His track record was good; so good, in fact, that doctors from several surrounding states referred patients—and sometimes their own wives—to him for the procedure. Indeed, Marcos Pupkin is most often described as "the doctor that other doctors send their wives to." Experience is an important part of any medical discipline, but in obstetrics, where one-third of the complications happen with no warning, experience is an extraordinarily valuable asset.

Dr. Pupkin is a smallish man with graying hair, glasses, and a soft, friendly South American accent reminiscent of Desi Arnaz. He received his MD from the prestigious University of Chile, and trained at the J. J. Aguerre Hospital in Santiago, which is not only one of the few hospitals in all of Chile but also one of the best hospitals in all of South America. He saw more than his share of complicated cases. Residents of Santiago have their babies there, but the peasants who live in the surrounding countryside have their babies at home, as they always have done, and they come to the hospital only when they know something is wrong. On an average day, young Dr. Pupkin and his fellow residents might delivery fifty babies, of which half a dozen might be complicated cases. An obstetrician in the United States may deliver a hundred babies before he sees a major complication; in Santiago, Pupkin saw them every day. By 1972, when he came to the United States for a two-year research fellowship at Duke University, he had delivered perhaps five thousand babies and presided over hundreds of complicated births.

The fellowship at Duke was for the study of maternal-fetal medicine—advanced obstetrics—and it was marked by two significant things. The first was the instant and enduring friendship that developed between Dr. Pupkin and Duke's director of maternal-fetal medicine, Dr. Carlyle Crenshaw. The other was a coup in Chile. In 1970, Chile's voters had elected Salvador Allende, a Marxist, to be president. By all accounts Dr. Allende was a moderate Marxist but as he began to nationalize U.S.-owned industries in Chile, the Nixon administration judged him a threat, and set about engineering his downfall.

Dr. Pupkin watched, from his vantage point in Durham, North Carolina, and thought about it. Living under a Marxist government did not appeal to him, but at least it was a popularly elected government. Then came the coup in 1973 and the military dictatorship of General Agosto Pinochet. A Marxist government might have been bad, Pupkin decided, but this was worse. When his two-year fellowship was over, Pupkin applied for and received a permanent faculty appointment at Duke. In 1977, he was granted U.S. citizenship.

Chile's loss was Carlyle Crenshaw's gain. Dr. Pupkin's vast experience was invaluable in any clinical obstetrics program, and Crenshaw was, by then, chief of clinical obstetrics at Duke. Pupkin later moved to Tulane University in New Orleans, but when Crenshaw began to assemble a team of obstetricians in 1980 to rebuild the University of Maryland's obstetrics department, his first phone call was to Marcos Pupkin.

Today, Dr. Pupkin is the number-two man in the department. He directs the clinical obstetrics program, he supervises the training of residents, and he runs the department in Dr. Crenshaw's absence. But most important, he serves as a reservoir of experience, a source of advice to his juniors and his peers alike. He cannot say precisely how many babies he has delivered in the last twenty-five years, but figuring the averages, it is probably something in excess of ten thousand. And that is the reason other doctors send their wives to him; no matter what happens, and no matter how suddenly it happens, Marcos Pupkin cannot be surprised. He cannot be caught off guard. He has seen it all.

[12]

Dr. Marcos Pupkin

DR. PUPKIN arrived in the ultrasound suite wearing a white lab coat over his scrub suit. He stood for a few moments outside the amnio room, looking at Laurie's ultrasound films, which were hanging on a lightboard, and talking in subdued tones with the radiologist. The radiologist pointed with a pencil as he recited all the normal findings the scan had disclosed. Finally, he pointed the tip of the pencil at a large dark spot on one of the films. Pupkin nodded approvingly.

The radiologist took down the films and placed them in a manila envelope. The two men had just turned and started toward the amniocentesis room when there was a commotion from one of the curtained-off ultrasound rooms. They heard a woman cry out, "No, no, oh God, no," and then break into sobs. Seconds later, an ultrasound technician burst through the curtains and looked around the outer room frantically. He spotted Pupkin and the radiologist and ran up to them.

"I need some help," he said to the two doctors. "This patient," he said, nodding his head toward the cubicle, "is so upset that I can't do the scans. She's crying so hard she can't hold still. Can you talk to her?"

Pupkin looked inquiringly at the radiologist. "She was here two weeks ago for amnio," the radiologist explained. "Her AFP was elevated and the original films showed what might have been a small meningocele, but we weren't sure, so we asked her to come back. I imagine that's why she's upset."

With the radiologist half a step behind him, Pupkin walked across the room to the cubicle, parted the curtain and walked in. A stocky, red-haired woman lay on the examining table, crying quietly; a man in work clothes stood beside her, holding her hand. As Pupkin entered, the man turned around and stared at him.

Pupkin's manner was friendly, but serious. "I'm Dr. Pupkin," he said. "I'm from the obstetrics department here. Is there anything I can do to help?"

"No—" the man began quietly, but his wife interrupted.

"I don't want this test," she sobbed. "I don't want it, I don't want it."

The man turned on her fiercely. "You have to have it," he snapped and was about to add something when Pupkin held up a hand. "Hold everything," he said, and the man stopped in midbreath. Like a good psychiatrist, Pupkin works consciously to put his patients at ease, but let the need arise and his voice can take on an edge that grabs the attention of whoever he is speaking to, and transmits the clear message that Professor Pupkin is in charge. Both the woman on the table and the man standing beside her stiffened, their eyes on Pupkin.

He held up a finger. "First," he said, looking at the woman, "if you don't want to have this test, nobody—" he glanced at the man. "You're her husband?" he asked. The man nodded. Pupkin looked back at the woman. "If you don't want the test, nobody, not even your husband, can force you to have it. If the two of you need time to discuss it, we'll find you a room where you can have some privacy.

"However," he continued, "before we do that, I want to make sure you understand that this is only an ultrasound exam. No needles today." He looked at the woman. "All we're doing today is taking another look at your baby."

The woman began to dissolve into tears again. Her husband looked up at Pupkin. "Can I talk to you?" he said. "I think I can explain."

"I think I understand," Pupkin said. "I know that your alpha fetoprotein test came back positive, and I'm sure that's what is worrying both of you. I have to tell you that we get a lot of false positives with that test. There may be nothing wrong at all, so we always want to double-check. That's why we want to do this second set of scans."

"That's not the whole story," the man said. "I had a brother with spina bifida. He was almost a vegetable. He couldn't walk, he was retarded, he couldn't talk, but he lived for nine years. I know what it's like to grow up in that kind of household. We've already got two kids, two fine, normal kids. I don't want to do that to them. Not even if it means giving up this baby.''

As Pupkin listened, he thumbed through the woman's hospital record. The couple's name was O'Malley. That figured, Pupkin thought. Every ethnic group carries its own peculiar genetic burden. Among blacks, there is sickle-cell anemia; Tay-Sachs disease is peculiar to Jews of Eastern European descent. Spina bifida, and associated neurological defects, occurs most frequently in persons of English-Irish ancestry. Finally, he found the radiologist's note describing the original ultrasound scans and glanced over it. There was a shadow on one of the images that could be consistent with a minor spinal defect, the note said. Reexamination was recommended. Pupkin looked up. ''From what I can see here,'' he said, ''we already know that this baby won't have anything as severe as your brother had. Anything that bad would have showed up on the first set of scans.''

The O'Malleys were watching him closely now. ''Let me explain a little bit to you about spina bifida. That's a term we don't use much because technically all it means is divided spine. You can have that and never know you have it. Where you get problems is when the spinal cord and the membranes around it are outside the spine. We call that myelomeningocele, and that's serious. We didn't see anything like that, did we?'' he glanced at the radiologist, who shook his head. ''We didn't see anything like that on the first scans.

''What we did see was a little shadow near the baby's spine. We don't know if it means anything or not. When the alpha fetoprotein test came back positive, we thought it would be a good thing to double-check.''

''Why do you need to double-check if you think the baby's okay?'' asked Mr. O'Malley.

''What I said was I don't think the baby has anything as severe as what you told me about your brother. The reason we want to check is to try to see if there's anything wrong at all. If there is, we want to be prepared for it when the baby's born.''

"I won't have to have an abortion?" Mrs. O'Malley asked thickly.

"No," Pupkin said quietly. "No, nobody can make you terminate a pregnancy if you don't want to. Sometimes we let people know it's an option, if we think it's the best thing, but we don't make the decision; you do."

"I just don't want a baby like my brother was," Mr. O'Malley said stubbornly.

"I don't think you have anything to worry about," Pupkin said, "but why don't we find out for sure right now?" He turned to Mrs. O'Malley. "Is it okay now? Can we have a look?" She nodded silently.

The ultrasound technician, who had been standing outside the curtain, slipped inside and went to his machine. He worked rapidly, as if afraid the woman might change her mind at any moment. The radiologist dimmed the lights, and the technician quickly began scanning across the woman's abdomen. When he located the baby's back, he began to hold the transponder very still, moving it slightly first one way and the another, highlighting, and capturing on film, the baby's vertebrae, starting at the head and moving down.

With its characteristic sounds the machine captured the vertebrae of the neck on film. A myelomeningocele that high on the spinal cord would be virtually untreatable; the baby, if it survived birth, would surely die soon afterward. But, the ultrasound clearly showed, the baby's neck was normal—unremarkable, in the jargon of radiologists. The upper back, around the shoulder blades, filled the next frame. It was normal. The rest of the thoracic vertebrae described a gentle curve on the screen, perfectly normal for a curled-up fetus. Next the lumbar vertebrae went on film, with no sign of malformation. Pupkin let out a long breath. The only parts left now were the sacrum and coccyx, and spinal defects there were not only rare, they were also usually reparable. These bottom vertebrae looked fine, too.

"There it is," Pupkin said to the couple. "As far as we can see, there's nothing to worry about. I'm sure that will make the next five months a lot more pleasant for you both."

Mrs. O'Malley raised herself on one elbow. "I'm sorry I was so much trouble," she said. Pupkin tried to dismiss her apology with a wave of his hand but she went on. "I didn't want to be so upset, but we're Catholics, and it would have been such an awful decision to have to make . . ."

"It's always an awful decision, no matter who makes it," Pupkin said quietly. "It's just that sometimes it's also the best decision. Just be grateful it's not a decision you have to make. Is everything okay now? I've got to go do some procedures."

Pupkin and the radiologist slipped out of the curtained enclosure and walked the short distance to the amniocentesis room.

Laurie lay on the table, her legs covered by a sheet, her hands clasped behind her head. Ann Jewell stood at the foot of the bed, Bill at the head. Pupkin nodded a greeting at Ann, then turned to Laurie. "Mrs. Edwards?" he said. Laurie nodded. "I'm Dr. Pupkin."

"Hi, Dr. Pupkin," Laurie said. "This," she added, nodding her head, "is my husband, Bill." The two men shook hands, then Pupkin turned back to Laurie.

"Sorry I made you wait so long," Pupkin said with a slight shrug. "We had a little crisis down the hall. Everything's fine now, but now I'm running even later than I expected."

"Don't get the idea that I'm too eager," Laurie said.

"How are you feeling?" he asked.

"Fine."

"Nervous?"

"Hell, yes," Laurie said with a wry smile.

"Good. If you weren't nervous, I would be," he said, bending to put two flat boxes on a storage shelf behind a stainless steel table and ripping open a third box to reveal an oblong, flat object wrapped in textured white paper. He placed that on the stainless-steel table beside the bed and opened the paper to reveal a white molded-plastic tray inside. "You know about the procedure now?" he continued.

"All too well," Laurie answered. "That's why I'm nervous."

"Well, we know there's a risk, but we think it's worthwhile.

You can still change your mind."

Laurie rolled her eyes back and glanced at Bill, then looking back at Pupkin. "No," she said. "I wouldn't want to waste all the worrying I've done."

As they spoke, Ann had adjusted the sheet and raised Laurie's gown, exposing her abdomen, and the radiologist had turned on the ultrasound machine. Then he squeezed a generous glob of the clear jelly onto the transponder and, as Ann turned down the room lights, pressed it against Laurie's abdomen.

Again, the room was lit by the eerie blue-gray glow, and all eyes focused on the monitor. This time Laurie saw what looked distinctly like a baby's face. Then the image shifted again. Pupkin and the radiologist pointed and conferred, pointed and conferred. The first consideration was to find a pocket of amniotic fluid as far from the baby's head and chest as possible. Pupkin's aim was accurate to within a few millimeters, but he liked to shoot for the largest target available, and that was one of the reasons his results were so good.

Next, they looked for any evidence of major blood vessels. A punctured artery or vein could contaminate the amniotic fluid with blood, making analysis difficult or impossible. More importantly, blood is an irritant. Too much of it and the uterus would begin to contract. It was usually impossible to stop such contractions, and sixteen-week preemies never survive.

That made it equally important to avoid the placenta, where maternal and fetal blood flowed past each other, separated by a one-cell thickness of membrane. There, the chances of puncturing an important blood vessel would be greater. Going through the placenta would double the risk. Sometimes that extra risk was tolerable, and in such cases Pupkin could usually get the needle safely through the minefield of blood vessels, but he preferred not to have to try. Happily, in Laurie's case the placenta lay in its usual place, along the back of the uterus. The pocket of amniotic fluid that showed on the ultrasound screen was at the top of Laurie's abdomen, near the baby's rump.

"There?" Pupkin asked, pointing to a dark area near the top of the screen.

"No, left a little," said the radiologist.

Pupkin moved his finger. "There?"

"Down."

"Right there?" Pupkin asked, still pointing.

"Right there," the radiologist answered. "About four centimeters down."

"That's a nice big one," Pupkin said admiringly.

"I told you," the radiologist answered. He lifted the transponder, pressed a finger against Laurie's abdomen, then, as the room lights came back on, moved the finger and pressed a tiny cone-shaped plastic object against her skin, right where the finger had been. He twisted it between his fingers briefly, then removed it. A tiny red circle remained.

"That's the target," Pupkin explained to Laurie as he turned back to the white plastic tray. "We've got a nice big pocket of fluid straight down from there."

Ann returned to the bedside and wiped the gel from Laurie's abdomen with tissue. Pupkin began pulling on sterile gloves. Ann threw the tissue into a trashcan, then took down a white plastic bottle of antiseptic from a shelf. She uncapped it and poured a tiny bit of it into the trashcan, a standard precaution that sterilized the neck of the bottle. Satisfied, she filled the one empty compartment in the white plastic tray with the dark-brown antiseptic. She capped the bottle and stepped back to the bedside, where she reached into a box and grabbed several syringes of various sizes, each one sealed inside a plastic tube.

Meanwhile, Pupkin busied himself at the tray briefly, then picked up a tiny, pink-handled sponge mop, dipped it into the antiseptic solution, turned, and began swabbing Laurie's upper abdomen with it. Three times he performed the scrub, then he reached for the sterile drapes.

"Are your hands comfortable?" Ann asked Laurie. "Once the drape's in place you won't be able to move them for a few minutes."

Laurie's hands were still clasped behind her head. She moved one hand and grasped Bill's. "Fine," she said.

There were two drapes, and they covered Laurie from her

chest to her thighs, leaving exposed only a tiny patch of skin with a fading red circle on it.

Pupkin lifted a glass ampoule of lidocaine, a local anesthetic, out of its plastic compartment, tapped it to move the bubble to the top, then broke the seal and set the ampoule upright in the tray. He shook a small syringe out of its sterile container, attached an inch-long needle to the syringe, dipped the needle into the lidocaine, and filled the syringe. That done, he twisted the needle off the end of the syringe and replaced it with a much smaller one.

"Everybody says this is the worst part," Pupkin said to Laurie as he turned back to the bed. "This is the local anesthetic, and it's gonna feel like a bee sting for a minute."

Holding the syringe almost horizontally, Pupkin slid the needle under the skin, so that the tip was beneath the tiny red circle, then moved the syringe slightly as he pushed the plunger, so the numbing fluid would reach as wide an area as possible. Laurie flinched and drew in her breath, but said nothing.

Pupkin turned back to the white plastic tray and lifted out a long, thin, plastic tube, twisted off the end, and withdrew a five-inch needle. He grasped it carefully between gloved thumb and forefinger, holding it parallel to his wrist as he moved it over the sterile barrier.

Laurie stared at the ceiling. It was a typical false ceiling, with white metal strips supporting rectangular acoustical tiles. The pattern on these tiles gave the impression of large wormholes interspersed with tiny, irregularly spaced pinholes. She selected a corner of one tile and started counting the pinholes, *one, two, three . . .*

Pupkin moved the point of the needle directly over the now-faint red circle on Laurie's abdomen. Holding his index finger over the top of the needle, he moved his thumb and second finger down the needle's shaft until they were four centimeters from the tip. Then with slow, deliberate downward pressure, he pressed the tip of the needle against Laurie's flesh.

Twenty-four, twenty-five, twenty-six . . . Laurie felt the pressure on her abdomen and held her breath, waited for the pinprick

sensation of the needle entering. *Twenty-nine, thirty, thirty-one*
. . .

The needle passed easily through the outer layer of skin,
down through the thin layer of fat beneath it, down, down,
straight down through three overlapping sheaths of connective
tissue, downward, a centimeter, two centimeters, three centimeters, to the hard, stretched, interlacing muscles of the uterus.

Thirty-four, thirty-five, thirty-six . . . Laurie had felt no pinprick, only pressure, an odd sort of pressure, not painful, not
even uncomfortable, really, but unpleasant nonetheless. It was
hard to tell exactly where the pressure was, but she could feel it
on the surface, and now she could feel it somewhere inside.
Thirty-nine, forty, forty-one . . .

Pupkin pushed harder on the needle, felt the stubborn uterine
muscle resist. Still holding the needle tightly, he pushed harder,
harder . . .

Forty-five, forty-six, forty-seven . . . now there was definite
pressure, uncomfortable pressure, somewhere inside, a cramping
feeling, getting worse, worse . . . *forty-eight* . . .

Suddenly the needle jerked downward until Pupkin's thumb
and second finger touched Laurie's skin. The needle was exactly
four centimeters deep.

Fifty, fifty-one, fifty-two . . . the cramp went away as quickly
as it had come, and Laurie let her breath out in a long, quiet sigh.
Pupkin straightened slightly and Laurie's eyes darted involuntar-
ily toward him. She caught herself, forced her eyes back to the
ceiling tile, too late. *Damn!* She'd lost her place. She drew in her
breath and started over, *one, two, three* . . .

Without loosening his grip on the needle, Pupkin removed his
index finger from the cap, and with his other hand he withdrew a
rigid stainless-steel wire, called a stylette, from the center of the
needle. The stylette fits snugly inside the bore of the needle and
prevents it from becoming clogged with cells as it moves through
the mother's flesh. Many early amniocenteses produced incorrect
results because the cells grown in culture turned out to be the
mother's cells, not the baby's. With the stylette out, a few drops

of clear liquid appeared at the top of the needle. Good. Perfect. Pupkin reached out his right hand, and Ann handed him a small syringe. With a quick twist he attached the syringe to the needle and pulled out the plunger. The clear, faintly yellow liquid filled the syringe. He twisted the syringe free, then turned to lay it on the sterile plastic tray as Ann handed him a much larger syringe. Pupkin attached it to the needle and pulled back the plunger, waited while it filled. Then another large syringe, then a small one. He filled the small one quickly and set it aside on the tray.

Forty-four, forty-five, forty-six . . . Laurie stared grimly at the ceiling. It didn't hurt, everything was fine, so why was she terrified? *Forty-seven, forty-eight . . .*

"Okay, that's it," Pupkin said. He grasped the shank of the needle with his right hand, pressed two fingers of the left against the skin around the needle, and with one swift motion pulled it straight up. A tiny bead of dark blood appeared at the spot where the needle had been, and Pupkin pressed an alcohol swab against it.

Forty-nine . . . as Laurie let go of Bill's hand, she realized that her own hand was dripping with sweat. She closed her eyes, let her head sink back against the pillow, and breathed deeply. Ann stepped forward to remove the sterile drapes.

Pupkin turned back to the white plastic tray and the syringes full of amniotic fluid. The first small syringe he ignored. Its purpose was merely to flush out any maternal cells that might have gotten into the needle despite the stylette. The other three, however, should be fine. One by one, he emptied their contents into three brown plastic test tubes with dark-brown screw caps. Then he handed them to Ann, who carefully wrapped them together with surgical tape, wrote "Edwards" on the tape, and stuck them in a pocket of her white lab coat.

The radiologist had disappeared during the procedure, so Pupkin took over the ultrasound machine himself, for one final scan. He knew that the procedure had gone perfectly and the likelihood of a complication with this one was minimal, but he always liked to reassure himself. Also, he liked to reassure the patient.

Applying more sterile jelly to the transponder, he pressed it against her midsection one final time. Ann dimmed the lights, and again Laurie could see the ghostly images of her unborn child. While she watched, Pupkin moved the transponder, and she could see the baby's heart beating.

"Good, good," Pupkin murmured as he stared at the monitor. "The baby looks fine."

[13]

In the Genetics Lab

IT WAS nearly one o'clock when Pupkin finished the last of the day's amniocenteses. There had been six of them, which was about normal, and five of them had been absolutely routine, but the last one had not gone well at all, by Dr. Pupkin's standards. The mother was fine, the fetus was fine, and the procedure had ultimately produced a satisfactory sample of amniotic fluid, but it had not gone with the smooth perfection Dr. Pupkin demanded of himself. The woman's placenta covered half the front of her uterus, and to avoid having to put the needle through the placenta, Pupkin had selected a pocket of amniotic fluid that the ultrasound scan showed to be in the upper left corner. The technician had marked it carefully, Pupkin had put the needle in equally carefully, he had successfully drawn off the first sample. Then the tap went dry, and no amount of jockeying could produce any more fluid.

Muttering under his breath, Pupkin had withdrawn the needle. The technician applied the transponder to the woman's abdomen, and sure enough, the pocket had moved. It happened sometimes. When the needle touched the outer surface of the uterus, sometimes it contracted slightly, shrank away, and squirted the fluid off in another direction like a bubble in a plastic bag of water.

Such a thing was not Pupkin's fault, but he had apologized abjectly and at length to the patient. Then he started all over again. The second time, the tap was perfect. He got the necessary 30 cc's of fluid and withdrew the needle, but as the tip of the needle came out, a tiny spurt of blood followed it. Cursing silently, Pupkin reached for a compress bandage. Inevitably, in a certain percentage of patients, the amniocentesis needle will puncture a tiny artery near the surface of the skin, and there will be more than the usual drop of blood. Moreover, some of the blood will leak into the tissue below the surface and will leave an ugly bruise-like discoloration that takes a few days to go away. Neither one of those events is remarkable, and certainly it is nothing serious, but it offended Pupkin's sense of proportion to have it happen to this particular woman, who had already had to endure being stuck twice with a needle.

He instructed her to press on the bandage for a few minutes, warned her that there might be a bruise, reassured her that it meant nothing, and did the final ultrasound scan. Apologizing again to the woman for the inconvenience, he left and stalked back to his sixth-floor office. For the rest of the day, he complained bitterly to anyone who would listen that it had been one of those days when *nothing* had gone right.

Meanwhile Ann Jewell, her pockets bulging with the six amniotic-fluid samples, made one last tour of the ultrasound suite, then headed for the elevators. She rode the elevator to the ninth floor, then walked briskly through a long maze of corridors and doors and across a covered bridge into the research tower adjacent to the hospital. She climbed two flights of stairs, walked down a hallway cluttered with lab equipment, arriving finally at a small laboratory marked CYTOGENETICS.

There were four women in white coats inside the lab; three of them stared intently into microscopes and made notes on lined tablets. The fourth sat at a long workbench, arranging two dozen clear-plastic tissue-culture flasks into six stacks of four each. There were murmured greetings as Ann walked in. ''How did it go?'' one of the technicians asked.

''Fine,'' Ann responded. ''We got all six.'' Sometimes patients changed their minds at the last minute, decided to think it over, decided not to have the procedure at all. Ann pulled a chair up to an empty stretch of workbench, took the six fluid samples out of her pockets, and arranged them carefully on the bench. Then she took out a sheaf of forms and started filling them out.

Amniocentesis is an extravagantly expensive procedure, because it requires a great deal of laboratory space, some very expensive equipment, and the time and attention of highly trained technicians. In teaching hospitals, some of that expense can be written off against research grants, and at the University of Maryland, much of the laboratory's initial start-up money came from the state health department. That meant there were a lot of forms to be filled out for each new amniocentesis performed. Ann worked steadily for a quarter of an hour, then finally gathered up all the forms and samples and handed them over to Joanne Beisel, the tissue-culture specialist.

It is not strictly necessary for a tissue-culture specialist to have advanced degrees in biology, and it is not strictly necessary for a tissue-culture specialist to know a great deal about human genetics; but Joanne Beisel does, and those things weighed heavily in her favor when she applied for the job. But what really mattered was that Joanne had had years of laboratory experience, was almost compulsively methodical in her laboratory technique, and, most important of all, understood the gentle and uncertain art of tissue culture.

As soon as it becomes attached to the uterine wall, the developing fetus begins to be surrounded by a membrane, and that membrane becomes filled with amniotic fluid. The fetus swims in the fluid, breathes it in and out of its developing lungs, swallows it, digests it, and excretes it. As those things happen, a few stray cells, mostly lung and skin cells, float away into the fluid. The cells are alive, capable of being grown in culture, and they carry the complete—and unique—DNA structure of the fetus that produced them. Each of the clusters of brown plastic tubes, bound together with surgical tape, was a living part of an unborn patient.

Joanne Beisel's first action after she received the fluid samples was to examine the forms and painstakingly prepare a series of labels for each patient, showing the patient's name, the case number, and the date. Four of the labels went onto the tissue-culture flasks, three more onto test tubes, with an extra wrapping of cellophane tape around the labels for good measure. An unlabeled fluid sample would be worthless.

A mislabeled sample would be worse. Much worse. Joanne had nightmares about mislabeled samples. As she wrote out the labels and stuck them onto the empty flasks and test tubes, she checked and rechecked the names on the forms. That task finished, she carefully entered each patient's name and number onto a separate page of a notebook. Then she double-checked the names again. There were horror stories about labs that mixed up two amniotic-fluid samples and discovered it three weeks later, when the cells were fixed onto microscope slides and a technician discovered two obviously different sets of chromosomes. If you were lucky, one would be a boy and the other a girl, so you'd know something was wrong and you could apologize to the patient and offer to do the procedure again. A few patients accepted, if it wasn't too late.

The worst case would be to mix up the cultures and see a case of Down's syndrome and tell the mother of a normal healthy fetus that the child would be born deformed. It would be horrible to reassure a worried mother that her baby was fine, only to have her deliver a defective one, but the absolute worst would be to erroneously tell a mother her baby was deformed, whereupon the woman would choose to have an abortion. Such cases were reported occasionally in the professional literature, and there were always rumors on the professional grapevine. That was why Joanne always double-checked, then checked again. It had never happened to her, and, she promised herself, it never would.

With the labeling finished, she threw a switch on the front of a large enclosed workbench, and a large fan roared to life. The sterile hood was equipped with a special ventilation system that blew sterile air from the back of the hood over the work surface so that no germs could come in from the outside air. And, in case the laboratory samples contained germs that should not reach the outside air, the air flow that passed over them was then sucked away to be resterilized. Sterility is the first requirement for successful tissue culture.

The next is a proper environment. It is the nature of most tissue cells to grow only when they are needed. If the skin is torn or burned, new cells grow rapidly to replace the damaged ones.

But when the growth is complete, it stops. Living, healthy cells that are surrounded by other living, healthy cells "know," through some exchange of chemical messages, that it is not necessary to divide. So the strategy of tissue culture lies in reproducing, in all the important details, the kind of environment that would make a single cell grow.

With the sterile hood activated, Joanne reached over to the workbench, picked up the first sample, and began unwrapping it. As soon as she got enough tape unwound to see the name "Edwards," she placed those tubes under the hood, turned, and selected the three test tubes also labeled "Edwards." She moved the three tubes to a holder inside the sterile hood, then resumed unwrapping the fluid samples.

Along with the three brown tubes there was a small clear-plastic syringe that also contained fluid. That was the first sample drawn, which was never used for tissue culture because sometimes it contained some of the mother's cells. Joanne had seen one case in which the lab predicted a girl and the mother delivered a boy. Obviously, the lab had cultured the mother's cells, not the baby's. So a new policy was instituted. Draw off a couple cc's of fluid to flush the needle; *then* collect the culture samples. But the first sample wasn't wasted. Joanne divided it into two small containers, and sent them off to two separate labs—more backup—to be checked for alpha fetoprotein.

For four hours, Joanne patiently gathered the cells from each of the six patients and divided each cell sample among four separate tissue-culture flasks. Finally, she fed them the laboratory equivalent of a high-calorie lunch, divided them into two groups, and put them into two separate incubators hooked to two separate power supplies. Nothing was left to chance.

Laurie and Bill had driven to the hospital in separate cars so they could go directly to work from the hospital. They had parked their cars beside each other in the underground garage, and after Laurie got dressed, they walked back to the garage together.

"You okay?" Bill asked, as they neared the automobiles.

"Yeah," Laurie said, letting out a long breath. "Yeah, I guess."

"Wanna have an early lunch?"

"I'm not really hungry. Bill, do me a favor."

"Sure."

"Call my office and tell them I'm not coming in, would you? I'm worn out. I'm gonna go home and take a nap."

Bill put an arm around her. "Want company?" he asked.

"Nah, you go to work. I'm just tired, that's all." She gave Bill a quick hug, got into her car and drove home.

As soon as she got there, she got in the shower and washed away the last of the dark brown antiseptic. Then, with minute care, she inspected the tiny wound at the top of her abdomen. She had seen the last ultrasound scan, had seen the baby's heart beating, and she knew that the baby was all right. But intellectual reassurance was worthless. She buttoned herself into a soft flannel nightgown, pulled down the shades in the bedroom, and lay silently in the darkened room.

Arguing before the Court of Appeals was a breeze compared to this. There you could do your research, make up your mind, take a position, and defend it. Legal questions, even when nitpicking, were clear-cut. Now she was in a situation where there were no right answers and there was too much advice. Laurie's Aunt Cindy had phoned three times in as many weeks; first to apologize and later to advise, then exhort, then beg Laurie not to have the amniocentesis at all. Now that it was done, Aunt Cindy would probably beg Laurie not to have an abortion no matter what the test results showed.

Laurie's mother and, for that matter, Bill's mother had been courteous, solicitous, and uncritical. Somehow, in Laurie's mind, that got translated to an even greater sort of pressure. They'd stayed in closer touch since they learned Laurie was pregnant, and every conversation began with an interrogation about Laurie's health. They meant well, but their exaggerated concern sent the unmistakable message: Worry. We hope you didn't wait too long, they were saying. We hope it's not too late.

Had she waited too long? The thought made her stomach churn. Had she been too materialistic, too ambitious, too selfish? What if it really was too late? She'd always known she wanted a child, and she'd always believed she'd have one, but events had conspired with one another, it seemed, to force her to postpone. She had achieved all her goals: Her marriage, her career, her life-style were as nearly perfect as twenty years of effort could make them; now she was fiercely determined to have the perfect pregnancy and the perfect child as well. And she was desperately afraid that she would fail.

Had she waited too long? Was it too late? She would know in three weeks, and to worry about it before then was futile, she told herself. It was done now, and there was no undoing it. She would, in due course, learn the results and, good or bad, she would have to live with them.

After a long time, the tears finally came. Then, exhausted, she fell asleep.

Bill came home from work early that afternoon, and he and Laurie spent a long, gloomy evening together. It was their tennis night, but neither one of them was in the mood. Instead they talked about the test, talked about what they would do if the results were bad.

"The first thing I'll do is get an unlisted telephone," Bill said sourly. He'd answered the phone two of the times Aunt Cindy had called. Laurie giggled at the thought; it was one of the few light moments of the evening.

Finally they both grew tired of the subject and agreed not to discuss it again until the results were in. There was no point in it; they had long since made all the decisions they needed to make.

Bill stood up and announced solemnly that he had decided to create a dish in honor of the occasion, a dish that would hence-forth be listed in all the great cookbooks of the world as "chicken amniocentesis." Laurie followed him into the kitchen and sat at the table while he cooked, which was probably a mistake, because it distracted Bill from his stove. While he was rubbing her shoulders a pan of shallots charred beyond redemption, and Bill burned two fingers rather severely when he sniffed the disaster and went lunging for the stove. Laurie finished cooking the chicken while Bill rubbed salve on his fingers. She hoped it wasn't an omen.

The next day, Laurie went back to work, and the first thing she found was a memo from the junior associate who'd handled the child-custody case. The case was open again and with a bizarre new twist: The mother and her boyfriend were petitioning to reopen the case, claiming that the boyfriend was the natural father of the children and that he and the mother were entitled to custody.

Laurie read the mother's formal petition to the court and whistled appreciatively. She'd been practicing law for fifteen years, and she'd never seen anything quite so diabolical. Not only was it the ultimate slap at the woman's ex-husband, it was also the sort of ploy that might cause a court to change its mind. This could be serious. Still reading the petition, she strolled out of her office and down to the law library, where she selected a thick volume of cases on the subject of paternity.

The work was a tonic for Laurie. It was probably the only thing that could have successfully moved her mind off the pending amniocentesis results. For nearly a week, her schedule returned to near-normal. She and Bill played tennis, and she won. They attended a party for one of Bill's coworkers who'd been promoted. Laurie drove to Annapolis to listen to one of the firm's junior partners argue his first case before a three-judge panel. She was absorbed in a law book when, a week after she'd had the procedure, her secretary buzzed the intercom. Ann Jewell from University Hospital was on the line, the secretary said.

Laurie's mind had been so far away that it took her a second to remember who Ann was. When she did, she panicked. It was too soon for results! This was the very thing Ann had warned her about! The only people who got quick results were the people with bad results! Her heart was pounding as her finger stabbed the flashing button on the phone. "How bad is it?" she asked without preamble.

Ann sounded slightly surprised. "Not bad at all," she replied. "In fact, it's very good. We got back the alpha-fetoprotein test results, and they're fine. I thought you might like to hear some good news."

Laurie let out a long breath. "I forgot about that," she confessed. "I thought you were calling with the other results, and I panicked because it was so soon."

Ann chuckled. "We're good, but we're not *that* good. Even bad results would take another week or so. I did check with the lab earlier today, though, and your cells are growing quite nicely. I'll probably call you again in about ten days with those results."

Laurie hung up the phone, went back to her book and read the same page three times before she gave up, slammed the covers shut, and stared at the wall. How the hell did she expect to be a competent mother if she panicked at every imaginary problem? She lectured herself. Grimly, she opened the law book.

Joanne Beisel heard about the good AFP test results from Ann Jewell; the outside labs always sent the results directly to Ann or Dr. Cohen, the division head. All six of the test samples had come back fine, which was good news. The lab people almost never saw the patients whose cells they cultured, but somehow they managed to become emotionally involved anyway. Bad test results always ruined everybody's day.

The day before, Joanne had wheeled a cart over to the incubator and had taken out forty-odd culture flasks. The secret of successful human tissue culture was to duplicate, as nearly as posible, the conditions of the human body. So the incubator maintained a temperature of exactly 98.6 degrees Fahrenheit, and a special gas bottle supplied extra carbon dioxide to the air inside the incubator. The nutrient solution contained a variety of chemicals, amino acids, growth hormones, even blood serum from calves, which was near enough to its human counterpart that skin cells didn't know the difference.

One by one, Joanne had placed the culture flasks on her microscope and examined them. All were doing satisfactorily. The cells tended to cluster together as they grew, and each flask, as she moved it around, showed promising numbers of cell clusters. It was also the nature of these cells to try to form a skin, and the clusters of cells had attached themselves to the bottom of the culture flask, which meant she could feed the cells.

Feeding the cells regularly was another part of the strategy to fool them into growing. Periodically the old nutrient solution was removed and replaced with fresh, creating the illusion of a circulatory system. For Joanne it was simply another painstaking job. Working under the sterile hood, she unscrewed the orange cap from a culture flask and with a single deft motion poured off the liquid. The cells clinging to the bottom of the flask, stayed in place. A glass pipette was already filled with nutrient solution, and she squirted the pink liquid into the flask, then replaced the cap so that the flask was exposed to the air for the shortest possible time. The cells were growing well; this certainly was not the time to risk any contamination.

When the small mountain of flasks had been fed, Joanne replaced them in the incubator and headed for the incubator in the next room. She was only half finished.

Laurie forced herself to concentrate on her books and papers, and by willpower alone was able to draw her attention away from the amniocentesis results. But whenever she relaxed her iron control, her thoughts would immediately shift and the dark fantasies of failure would intrude again. For some reason, the most persistent image was of the abortion she would have to have. She imagined lying on an examining table in a very cold room while masked, hooded figures performed nameless and unspeakable acts, hidden from her view by a bedsheet. It was sheerest nonsense, she knew: Second-trimester abortions were performed by inducing premature labor. She'd read all about it in her textbook. It would be like having a baby, only not as painful; at least not physically. But the torture-chamber image persisted. Once or twice she had nightmares about it.

Bill must be going through the same things, she knew, even though they were carefully not discussing it with each other. But they'd been going to plays and concerts at least once a week, sometimes twice. That, she knew, was Bill's way of distracting himself.

One tennis evening they decided, instead of playing, to bundle up and go for a walk instead. For nearly an hour they wandered up and down the back streets of their neighborhood, saw houses they never knew were there, and amazingly enough, they carried on a spirited conversation that had nothing to do with pregnancy or abortion. When they got back to the house, Laurie made hot chocolate while Bill built a fire, and they snuggled in front of the fireplace sipping their steaming cocoa, and agreeing that they should take more walks.

Then the baby moved.

"Jesus!" Laurie whispered, and she sat bolt upright, almost spilling her cocoa. "Quick, gimme your hand. Feel." She grabbed Bill's hand, held it against her. The baby obligingly moved again.

"Omigod," Bill said quietly. "Does that mean something's wrong?"

"No, dummy, that means the baby's fine. That's what's called quickening. That was the first time it happened."

Bill held his hand on her abdomen until the baby moved again. "Well, I'll be damned," he said. Then he paused, and added quietly, "But I sort of wish he'd waited until after . . ." The sentence trailed off.

"So do I," Laurie replied. They sat for a while, staring at the fire, saying nothing. Laurie's mind was strangely calm. She regarded the event as a good omen; somehow she was certain now that the baby was fine.

[14]

Results

WAITING for the amniocentesis results proved, as everyone had predicted, to be the toughest part of the entire procedure for Laurie. For the first time, law books failed to hold her attention. She could concentrate for a while, but some stray phrase, often only a single word, would trigger the thoughts again, and a few minutes later she'd catch herself woolgathering. The reopened child-custody case languished. In a brief court appearance, Laurie had argued that the case deserved slow, cautious, careful study, and the judge had agreed, scheduling a formal hearing the following month.

She began reading the textbook again. Finding it was not difficult at all; Bill had concealed it behind several large cans of paint, in the same cupboard where he'd once hidden her cigarettes in an attempt to get her to quit smoking. It was the first place she looked for the book. Bill, she reflected affectionately, sometimes showed a startling lack of originality.

Reading the book couldn't possibly hurt now, she decided. Nothing she could find in the book could cause her any more anxiety than she already was going through. She put the book in her briefcase and took it to her office where, during the next week, she read it from cover to cover.

On Friday of the seventeenth week of her pregnancy, Laurie left work early; but instead of going home, she drove to the offices of Drs. Bennett and Bennett, dentists. As soon as she'd found out that Norma Bennett's amniocentesis results were good, she'd called and made an appointment to have her teeth cleaned. It was something she'd needed to have done for a while; she figured it would be efficient to combine that with a gossip session.

She was the last patient on the schedule, which was deliberate. It gave her a natural exit, or, if the conversation was going well, a natural opportunity to invite Dr. Bennett to continue the chat over a glass of wine.

She arrived to find Dr. Bennett in the waiting room, sitting sideways on a love seat, with her feet propped up on one armrest.

"I've spent most of the last twenty years on my feet," she complained. "You'd think they'd be used to it by now. I wear good shoes and support hose, and they *still* hurt. And now that I'm carrying around all this extra weight," she said, patting her middle, "they hurt even more."

The informality was contagious. Laurie sat down on a love seat next to Dr. Bennett's, kicked off her shoes, and drew her feet up under her. "I guess I'm lucky," she said. "I work sitting down."

"I envy people like you sometimes," Dr. Bennett replied. "But I suppose I'm better off getting the exercise. What do you do for exercise now that you're pregnant?"

"I still play tennis, but slowly," Laurie said. "I'm going to give it up soon. This," she said, pointing to her middle, "makes me off-balance, and I'm always afraid I'm going to fall on it. I'm going to have to find something easier, I suppose."

"Did you get your results yet?" Dr. Bennett asked abruptly.

Laurie shook her head. "That's one reason I'm here. I guess I need some reassurance."

"Don't look at me," Dr. Bennett said in mock horror. "I'm a dentist. I *cause* pain. Do you want to ruin my image?"

Laurie chuckled. "You reassure me just by being two months ahead of me, and having everything go well for you. I was almost as thrilled as you were when I hard your results were good."

Dr. Bennett beamed. "Yeah," she said, "yeah. We didn't even celebrate until the next day. I just went home and cried. I was so relieved. We had already talked about adopting, on the assumption that this—" she patted her middle again "—wouldn't work out. I really didn't think it would; my God, I'm almost forty-five years old. You can't imagine what a relief it was. And a boy, too, on top of everything else—Jason McWhirter Bennett the third," she said proudly. Abruptly, she swung her feet around and stood up. "Back to business," she said. "C'mon. Follow me. We can talk while I do your teeth."

Dr. Bennett led Laurie down a short hallway to a room with a chaise-lounge-style dentist's chair, richly padded and covered with what looked to Laurie like real leather. It was the only luxurious item in an otherwise spartan room; Laurie glanced around at the cabinets, x-ray machines, lights, cables, and the inevitable chairside utility tower, complete with a pastel blue porcelain spit sink. The only article on any of the walls was a translucent lightboard for examining X rays. Laurie sat down tentatively on the leather chair, then swung her legs up and leaned back. It was, she reflected, out of character to have such a comfortable chair in a dentist's office.

The dentist selected a handful of items from a multi-drawered cabinet, then walked over to the chair and laid the items on the circular stainless steel table. She adjusted the overhead light, rearranged the instruments on the circular table, then picked up the one with a tiny mirror at its end. "Let me look around a bit first," she said. Laurie obligingly opened her mouth.

"The most amazing thing about doing this while you're pregnant," Dr. Bennett began without fanfare, "is that the baby never kicks. It's like he knows. When I take a break and sit down, sometimes he kicks the breath out of me, but he's always very considerate of my patients.

"I worried about that the first time I was pregnant, which was . . . jeez, Kimberly is twelve now, so I guess that was thirteen years ago. Talk about feeling old." As she talked, she moved the mirrored instrument throughout Laurie's mouth, stretching lips and cheeks to get a look at the far sides of her teeth. "Mac and I—Mac's my husband—worried about that, and I thought about just stopping work for the last four or five months, but I would've gone nuts. Finally, we decided that I'd stick with cleaning teeth, not do any fillings or anything. But then it turned out that the baby stays quiet while I'm on my feet. It's amazing. I don't know why that is, but it's been true every time now."

"Mnnng," Laurie murmured. She wanted to tell Dr. Bennett that she had experienced her own "quickening" only the week before, but the dentist continued to explore Laurie's mouth.

"You've got a cavity back there," Dr. Bennett said, tapping Laurie's lower left molars with the mirror. "It's a little one. Looks new. It's not very deep. You ought to get it filled right away." She withdrew the mirror. "Other than that, your teeth are in amazingly good shape. They don't really need cleaning. I'm just going to polish them for you."

"How bad a cavity?" Laurie asked, exploring the tooth in question with her tongue.

"It's very small," the dentist replied, snapping a tiny brush attachment onto the drill mechanism. "You could probably go for months and not get a toothache from it. But the sooner you get it filled, the easier it will be. Okay, open wide now." She dipped the brush into a tiny container of tooth polish, pressed it against Laurie's upper front teeth and stepped on a switch. The brush grew hot as it ground against Laurie's teeth. The abrasive paste, she noted, was orange-flavored.

"Anyway," Dr. Bennett said, "Little Mac—what a family! The men are Big Mac and Little Mac—started kicking right on schedule. You know, it's a little strange, knowing that I've got a boy, and here I've got almost three months to go. It gives him a sort of personality. That's something that's different from my first two; both of them were surprises. Okay, rinse your mouth out." As Laurie rinsed, Dr. Bennett asked, "Have you thought about whether you want to know? They give you the choice, you know."

"I know. I don't want to know. I want to be surprised," Laurie replied.

"I think you're right," the dentist said. "Open a little wider . . . " she began polishing Laurie's lower teeth. "I got the best news I could possibly get, of course, that everything was fine, and that it was a boy besides, but I've thought about it, and I don't know how I'd feel if it was a girl. We really did want a boy, and I think I'd have been disappointed, and I don't know if that's healthy. When you have three or four months to think about it *before* you deliver, it can change the way you feel about the baby *after* you deliver. I think if I had it to do again, I wouldn't want to know. It's better that way. We were hoping for a boy when we had Wendy, but when they handed her to me it was such a thrill, there's nothing like it. Open wider . . . you're closing up on me.

"I wish there was something I could tell you that would make you not worry," she went on, "but I'd be silly to try. I was just sick with worry for those three weeks, and really for the whole first part of the pregnancy, because of what happened before. Okay, rinse again."

"How did you find out, that time?" Laurie asked when her mouth was clear. She had hoped for a chance to ask just that question; it was one of the reasons she had come. Her fantasies of receiving bad news had reached such awful proportions that they had blended into her nightmares, and now she half-expected a knock on the door at midnight by a somber messenger in a black uniform.

"Oh, Ann phoned," Dr. Bennett said. "Open a little wider, please. I'm almost done. Ann phoned. It was very straightforward. She just said 'I'm afraid I've got bad news; the test shows that the baby has Down's syndrome.' And that was it. She was very nice. She called on a Tuesday, and I went in the hospital the next day, two weeks after the amnio. You can rinse again now."

The cool water felt good in Laurie's mouth; her teeth tingled from the pressure of the polishing brush. She swirled the water past her teeth, spat it into the little bowl, and sat back. Dr. Bennett was rearranging the instrument tray.

"You want me to fill that cavity right now?" she asked. "It'll take about ten minutes, it's so small. I hate to think you came all the way over here just to have me brush your teeth."

"I didn't. I also came to talk. I'd have gone to Philadelphia to talk, if that's where you were. I've been going nuts; I don't know any pregnant people to talk to, and especially not people who've gone through what you've gone through, and what I'm going through."

Laurie paused, thought a moment. "How long did you say I could go before that cavity will give me trouble?"

"Six months, a year. A long time. But the longer you wait the bigger filling you'll need."

"How about I come back in a couple weeks? I'm sure you'll want to hear my good news."

"Deal. I'm sure you'll have good news to tell, too. I bet you'd have heard by now if it was bad." Dr. Bennett snapped off the examining light, and began putting the dental instruments in a stainless steel container.

Laurie sat still in the dentist's chair. "I don't want to pry, but I'm so scared that I'll have to have an . . . abortion." She forced herself to pronounce the word. "I know it can't be as bad as I imagine it. How do they do it?"

Dr. Bennett busied herself at the instrument cabinet. She looked at the wall as she spoke. "They induce labor," she said quietly. "They give you vaginal suppositories of prostaglandin, and in a few hours you go into labor and deliver. It's much easier than labor at term, not as painful, doesn't take as long. It was so sad. I finally gave up and asked them for a Valium, and I *never* take tranquilizers. That's how sad it was.

"But it was the right thing to do," she said, her voice firming. She turned around. "After I got the Valium in me I got so calm that I told them I wanted to see it, and they brought it in, and even I could tell that it would've been horrible. The head was all out of shape. It would've had Down's syndrome, and hydrocephalus, and later they told me it would've had heart defects, too. It was sad, but I've never regretted it for a minute, and of course now," she said, patting her middle, "now I've got little Mac here, and I know he's fine. I'd say it was a fair trade."

"Yeah," Laurie said distantly. "Yeah." Her mind was racing. Such a simple solution! Why hadn't she considered it in all her bleak scenarios of disaster? Of course she would get pregnant again, right away. It would make the tragedy bearable, turn a nightmare into a fair trade. Why hadn't she thought of that before?

"You want me to schedule you for that filling right now?" Dr. Bennett asked.

"Nah," Laurie said, "My calendar's a real disaster for the next couple weeks. Better let me dicker with your secretary."

It is not inaccurate to call the optical devices in the genetics lab "microscopes," but it is an understatement amounting almost to injustice, like calling a Rolls Royce "a car," or chateaubriand "food." These instruments are manufactured by the Zeiss works in Germany, and contain some of the most precisely ground lenses and prisms in the world. The special high-power lenses are so finely aligned that they have to be filled with a special clear oil to avoid distorting the light waves as they pass from lens to lens. The precision optics are matched by a set of ultraprecise indexing controls that give each spot on the slide its own unique address. And when a noteworthy specimen is located, a built-in camera can record it on 35mm film at the touch of a button. The devices are indeed microscopes, but at thirty-seven thousand dollars apiece they are hardly ordinary.

The genetics lab has three of the microscopes and three technicians who spend long, tedious hours staring into them, examining the slides that Joanne Beisel prepares. The process of examining, identifying, and cataloging chromosomes is called karyotyping, and to become expert at it requires many months, sometimes even years. To the untrained eye, the chromosomes that lie amid the ruins of a shattered skin cell look like little more than a cluster of fuzzy black dots. With experience, it becomes possible to identify individual chromosome pairs by comparing them to charts showing each pair's unique shape and staining characteristics. The technicians who examime these cells after day become so adept at it that when they look at the tangled mass of chromosomes, an abnormality will fairly leap through the lens at them.

In a less formal place, the technician might simply glance over a slide or two, assure herself that the chromosomes look normal or abnormal, and send a memo to the doctor, who would notify the patient. Ninety-nine times out of a hundred, they would be absolutely accurate. But in the field of genetics, where unborn lives are at stake, ninety-nine percent accuracy is not enough. The first few chromosome clumps told the technician everything she needed to know about the patient, but lots of other people would want to check her results. So as she twirled the indexing knobs and located cluster after cluster of chromosomes on the slide marked "Edwards," she captured the two or three best ones on film.

A day or two later, a stack of black-and-white photographic prints showed up on the microscope bench, and the day after that, the technician located a second trio of slides marked "Edwards," which she dutifully examined and photographed. The slides went back into a storage tray in the lab, and the film was sent to the darkroom.

When the second set of prints arrived in the lab, the technician selected the two best ones with the name "Edwards" on them, sat down with a pair of surgical scissors, and began cutting out the individual chromosomes like so many tiny paper dolls. She carefully matched them into pairs and pasted them onto a prepared form. The two forms, when completed, showed two identical sets of twenty-three chromosome pairs.

The technician slipped the two sheets, along with the spare prints, into the file folder labeled "Edwards," moved the folder to the stack marked "completed," and reached for the next set of photographs.

On the Wednesday of the eighteenth week of her pregnancy, Laurie dutifully reported for her regular examination, carrying the obligatory olive jar full of early-morning urine. She still thought the process was an annoyance, but she'd learned enough about the reasons for the annoyance to be more than willing to endure it. If she had been confronted, Laurie would have denied that the fear of having a less-than-perfect pregnancy made her anxious, even eager, to be examined as often as possible; instead, she would have argued that now she simply knew more about the nature of the exam and the reasons for doing it, and that made it more tolerable.

Dr. Crenshaw was chatty and amiable, but his eyelids drooped with fatigue. He'd been on call the night before, he said, and had delivered two babies. He ushered Laurie into an examining room and reappeared almost as soon as she was undressed and installed on the table. He examined her abdomen thoroughly, pressing it gently with his fingertips, and sometimes with both hands. He used a tape measure to determine the distance in centimeters from her pubic bone to the top of her bulge, and made a note of the number. And he did a ten-second pelvic exam using only his fingers.

Laurie endured it all with good grace. She knew now that when he palpated her belly he was verifying what the ultrasound exam had shown, that the baby was in the normal head-down position. If the baby seemed to have changed position, it would mean Laurie would require close watching as she approached the end of her pregnancy. If the baby was in any position other than the head-down "vertex" position when she went into labor, then Laurie would probably be delivered by cesarean section. Study after study had showed that while breech babies could often be delivered safely through the vagina, they could more often be delivered more safely by cesarean section.

Crenshaw chatted casually with Laurie during the examination, and he seemed delighted to hear that the baby had begun moving. That had happened right on schedule, he said. Laurie paid close attention to Crenshaw's reactions as he examined her. As long as his manner remained casual, she had concluded, she had no cause for alarm. If he suddenly got very quiet, and seemed very interested in something, then she would worry.

The tape measure, she knew, told Crenshaw the correct fundal height. Measuring the distance from the pubic bone to the fundus, or top of the uterus, is one of the oldest diagnostic tricks known to obstetrics, and will likely remain a staple of the business for as long as obstetrics endures. Starting at about the eighteenth week of pregnancy, and continuing on through about the thirtieth week, the number of centimeters between the two points is approximately equal to the number of weeks of gestation. A significant variation, one way or the other, is sufficient reason to order up a battery of more sophisticated tests to find out why. Laurie didn't see the number he wrote down, but she remembered from the ultrasound exam two weeks before that the baby was the proper size.

The vaginal exam, she knew now, was to check her cervix, to be sure it was intact. It was at about this stage of pregnancy that an incompetent cervix would begin to give way. If that happened, the cervix would feel much shorter than before, and very quickly, probably the same day, Crenshaw would move Laurie to the obstetric operating room, where he would anesthetize her and sew her cervix closed with strong black silk thread. Laurie had read in her textbook that there were two methods of cerclage, as the book called it. Both methods were effective treatments for an incompetent cervix, and were named for their inventors, Shirodkar and MacDonald. Her text seemed to favor the Mac-Donald stitch, and had Crenshaw suddenly become interested as he examined her cervix, she would have asked about the relative merits of the two different stitches. But Crenshaw withdrew his fingers after only a few seconds, and Laurie knew that meant he'd found only what he expected.

Laurie dressed quickly after the exam, then went next door to the consultation room, where Crenshaw sat reading Laurie's record. He congratulated her on her excellent progress so far, up to and including the good alpha-fetoprotein test results. Laurie admitted guardedly that she was, well, somewhat anxious about the amniocentesis results and wondered aloud if there was any way of estimating how much longer it would take. Crenshaw consulted the chart. "I would say that if the results were bad, very probably you would have already heard about it," he replied.

"That, of course, is not a guarantee," Laurie interposed.

"That is not a guarantee," Crenshaw agreed, "but once again we are talking about probabilities. The longer it takes for you to get results, the greater the probability that the results will be good. But to answer your original question, you surely ought to hear something within the next week or ten days.''

It was a terrible way to spend a pregnancy, Laurie complained bitterly to herself. It was three weeks since the amniocentesis and still no results, and that, she had to remind herself doggedly, was a good sign. To be a lawyer requires a special sort of mental discipline and again and again Laurie used that iron will to fight her natural anxiety. Laurie was desperately afraid and no amount of logic, no amount of lecturing herself, no amount of evidence would convince her that the worries were unfounded. Not, at least, until the amniocentesis results were in.

She forced herself to concentrate on her work, which at the moment consisted largely of reading, and approving or rewriting, several incredibly complex corporate merger proposals. Laurie had become the law firm's antitrust expert, at first simply because she was the only one who had the patience to actually read the contracts, cover to cover. She understood them, remembered them, and remembered all the laws and court rulings that applied, which quickly earned her the reputation of a genius in the field. Then she had defended and won a couple of spectacular cases, so that now the word had begun to spread, and larger and larger corporations had begun approaching her firm for advice.

And if those cases were unexciting, there was always this child-custody case. Laurie had claimed that one for her own, and when the beleaguered father had come to her on the verge of tears and confessed that he had no money with which to pay her, she had immediately told him that she wouldn't charge him for her services. She knew she was going to have a lot of fun when they got into court. She hadn't had been to a good old-fashioned courtroom brawl in years. This was definitely going to be one, and she was going to win it.

The baby kicked and a tiny wisp of panic raced around the fringes of her mind hissing fearful thoughts: it was too late; she'd waited too long, she would fail, she had blown it.

Laurie had wondered once or twice whether the fear she felt

was because she loved the baby inside her, or because she was such an egomaniac that she couldn't bear the thought of failure. It was an uncomfortable question. There were times when she felt great tingling surges of love for this unborn child, times when she would fantasize about the delivery, which would be perfect, of course, and about seeing her daughter for the first time, who would be perfect too, of course. Then the fantasy leaped ahead in time, to a quiet room with lace curtains that softened the sunlight, where she would breastfeed her baby, awash in love and serenity.

There were the nightmares as well. In the great stone dungeonlike room stern, disapproving men would disappear behind the bedsheet and carry away her baby in a bucket. Once or twice the nightmares visited the delivery room, where everything was fine until the moment the baby was born, and then suddenly everyone became quiet, and there was no sound, no baby crying, and one by one the people silently left the room until Laurie was there alone.

She'd talked it over with Trish Payne, who'd assured her that both sorts of fantasies were perfectly normal; that indeed they were common to most pregnant women. She noted the logic of that, but persisted in feeling guilty about the failure fantasies. Perhaps they were an expression of subconscious wishes, she thought. Perhaps she *wanted* to fail. Perhaps she didn't love the baby enough. Perhaps she wasn't capable of love anymore. Perhaps it really was too late.

Three weeks and two days after the amniocentesis, Ann Jewell opened the file folder marked "Edwards," glanced over the report, and picked up the telephone.

If anyone understands the intensity with which a mother can worry about her unborn baby, Ann Jewell does. She is the mother of twins, and a pregnancy with twins is always considered a high-risk pregnancy, for both the mother and the babies. Preeclampsia, although it is rare, strikes women carrying twins more often than mothers with single babies. Packing two babies into a space intended for one can cause problems by itself, up to and including the ultimate horror of Siamese twins.

But that was only the beginning. Ann is a trained geneticist, and although she knew her family tree was free of danger signs, she also understood that a certain number of genetic defects occur without warning, spontaneously. And she understood fully just how many different birth defects there are; entire books are devoted to the description and classification of birth defects.

Ann is still in her twenties, well below the age at which doctors will recommend amniocentesis. Still, she says, she might have considered having the procedure, simply for the reassurance it would have provided. But even that door was closed to her, because she had twins. With twins the uterus is so crowded that there is no margin for error, and except in the most extreme cases, obstetricians will not perform amniocentesis on women with twins. The risk is simply too high.

A tertiary-level hospital like the University of Maryland attracts patients from all along the Eastern Seaboard because it has the equipment and staff of experts necessary to treat the rarest and most severe medical problems. The odds against the occurrence of some of them are hundreds of thousands or even millions to one, but they do happen, and Ann has seen many of the extremely rare, and extremely severe, birth defects that can occur. During the entire nine months of her own pregnancy, she worried about them. She knew it was irrational and unreasonable to worry, but she worried anyway, and her work as a geneticist gave her an endless supply of things to worry about. Ann ultimately delivered two perfectly normal, healthy twins. But she understands, in exquisite and personal detail, the nature of prenatal anxiety.

In moments of great stress, the mind stretches time. From the instant a mother realizes that this will be The Phone Call until the time Ann can deliver the news is an eternity, an agony of panic, of doubt, of anxiety. Ann knew that, and tailored her opening remarks accordingly. When Laurie answered, Ann said, in a single breath, "Hi, this is Ann, it's good news, everything looks fine."

Across town, Laurie leaned back in her swivel chair and let out a long breath. "Wonderful," she said. "Wonderful."

"I've got the charts in front of me," Ann went on, "and everything's normal. We don't see anything that would cause us to suspect any genetic problems."

Laurie brushed at a tear, then giggled in relief. She had rehearsed all sorts of responses to bad news; now she was all but speechless. "You know what the worst part is?" she finally asked.

"What?" Ann replied.

"The worst thing is that I can't even go out and get drunk to celebrate, 'cause I'm pregnant."

Ann chuckled. "You're right. You can celebrate all you want about four months from now. I have one question for you: Have you changed your mind about wanting to know the baby's sex?"

Laurie thought about it again for a moment. For a brief instant, she conjured up the fantasy of the sunlit room, and the infant was a daughter. What if it were a son?

"No," she finally answered. "No, let me hang onto my fantasies a while longer."

[15]

Dr. Norma Bennett

LAURIE'S PREGNANCY, and indeed her whole life, seemed to divide into two epochs: before the amniocentesis and after the results. The time in between was a sort of limbo—later she had only the faintest recollection of actual events. She remembered that the baby had begun moving during that time, and she remembered going for long walks with Bill, and she remembered being examined by Dr. Crenshaw; but those were isolated events, tiny unconnected patches of memory in a great emotional fog.

She felt ashamed, intellectually, for not having beaten back the terror, for having been unable to banish it with logic. Any reasonable person would have known that the odds were on her side and wouldn't have worried so intensely. She was, in retrospect, proud of herself for having confessed her terror only to Dr. Bennett. Lawyers were supposed to be tough; somehow, she had managed to hang onto that image around most people. Still, she was entitled to worry, she reminded herself. Everyone had told her that. She was *supposed* to worry a little bit. It proved she cared about her baby. She would resume worrying in due course, she thought, smiling to herself. Now that she *knew* things were all right, she felt only an overwhelming sense of relief, and she planned to wallow in it awhile.

The twenty-two-week checkup was indistinguishable from the one before it. Crenshaw felt her abdomen, measured it, and announced that everything was fine. They chatted briefly, and Crenshaw assured Laurie that she was making perfectly satisfactory progress.

The baby kicked, and Laurie smiled beatifically down at her bulging middle. She had tried hard to keep her emotional distance from the baby while abortion was still a possibility, had failed, and felt guilty for even trying. Now there were no self-imposed barriers, and she let the warm tides of emotion wash over her. She was sure it was a girl. She fretted over not knowing something that other people knew and more than once Laurie had reached for the phone to call Ann Jewell and find out. If it was a boy, she would love it and pamper it and cherish it and raise it as Bill's son, his heir. But in all her fantasies it was a girl, *her* girl, a devoted daughter who would be beautiful, feminine, brilliant, the class valedictorian *and* the homecoming queen.

More and more now, her fantasies turned toward the delivery itself. She had been unable to consider it before, knowing that, at twenty weeks, an abortion would have been perversely similar to labor and delivery at full term. Now that she expected to carry the baby for the remaining twenty weeks, she was free to consider, in her reveries, the act of childbirth. She was curiously ambivalent about it. She knew it would be painful, messy, ignoble, and a dozen other unpleasant things, yet somehow she looked forward to it. She'd read and reread the section in her textbook about "parturition," but it was like reading about sex; no amount of academic knowledge could substitute for experience. She was looking forward to attending childbirth classes; Trish Payne had promised that by the end of the classes there would be no surprises left for the delivery room.

Her middle had begun to swell rapidly now. Before, she had been obviously pregnant; now she was getting huge. She had been gaining weight at about two and a half pounds per month for the first four months; now the rate accelerated to three and a half pounds. She mentioned it to Dr. Crenshaw when she went for her checkup at twenty-two weeks; he replied that it was about time for that.

The day after she'd gotten the amnio results, she phoned Norma Bennett's office. Dr. Bennett was unavailable, but Laurie left a message with the secretary. She'd sought out Dr. Bennett so she could talk about amniocentesis and abortion, but after chatting with her, she found she enjoyed the dentist's informal, matter-of-fact air. Besides, there were few enough women Laurie could talk with about all the perils and travails of pregnancy. Most of her friends had teenagers now, and a few had grown children, and they were always faintly patronizing when Laurie tried to describe experiences that, to her, were fresh and new.

Laurie and Bill continued to take long strolls through the neighborhood. It was relaxing and invigorating, and Laurie was no longer in the mood for tennis. Her back had begun to ache, which was not surprising, considering that she was now almost twenty pounds heavier. Oddly, the walking seemed to help.

The baby, Laurie imagined, seemed to enjoy the walks. It stayed very quiet when they walked, but afterward, when they'd sit in front of the fireplace, the baby seemed almost to grow restless, and would shift around repeatedly, as though complaining that the gentle rocking motion had stopped. Bill seemed fascinated by the movements, and would sit, motionless, with his hand on Laurie's belly. Those were quiet, golden moments; they rarely spoke, and rarely needed to. Laurie often fantasized about what life would be like after she had the baby. She tried to imagine taking the child with her to the office, and somehow the fantasy never seemed quite right. There was no place for babies inside stuffy old law firms. She decided she'd do it once, and that would be it. Soon the fantasy shifted to her favorite, the one where she stood behind lace curtains, bathed in soft light, and nursed her child.

Bill, whose carpentry skills—and power tools—had languished since they'd finished the house, had begun building a cradle. He complained halfheartedly about not knowing whether to build a boy-crib or a girl-crib, and growled when Laurie suggested with a straight face that he build a unisex one.

Meanwhile, they'd been slowly consolidating their two studies into one, emptying out the room next to their bedroom. That room had been Bill's study, and they had chosen it for the nursery. It had the twin advantages of being adjacent to their own bedroom and of having less junk in it. Bill brought home work less often than Laurie, and his study was more like a television room, where he sometimes retreated to watch football games.

Laurie's study, on the other hand, was littered with books, papers, court documents, transcripts, and law-review magazines. Laurie spent a great deal of time straightening up her own mess in order to make room for Bill's stuff. It took them several weekends to do it, but they finally emptied the nursery-to-be. Bill promised to buy paint, and Laurie began consulting her decorator catalogs for furniture ideas.

Three days before her twenty-six-week checkup, Laurie consulted her calendar, then phoned Bill from work and suggested they have dinner in Baltimore's Little Italy that night. Dr. Crenshaw had told her to be sure to eat larger-than-normal amounts of pasta, cake, confections, and other sinful things for a few days before her checkup. She spent the afternoon salivating as she thought about fettucine Alfredo.

The twenty-six week checkup was not materially different from the twenty-two week checkup; but, on instructions, Laurie had eaten no breakfast that morning. Dr. Pupkin was filling in for Dr. Crenshaw that day, and he checked all the same things with the same professional aplomb that Laurie had begun to watch for; you don't worry unless the doc suddenly gets interested.

Before the exam, Pupkin explained the diabetic screening test to her. Diabetes, he reminded her, sometimes occurs spontaneously in pregnant women, even in women who have no history of diabetes and whose blood sugar levels have remained relatively normal throughout the early parts of the pregnancy. Laurie had, up to this point, been completely normal, but to be absolutely safe, they now wanted to put stress on her insulin system to see how well it worked.

The reason she'd been told to load up on sweets and starches for a few days was to be sure that her pancreas, which secretes insulin, had been working steadily for a few days. The results were more consistent and more meaningful that way. All she had to do now was to drink this little bottle of sweet stuff, wait an hour, and let a nurse take a blood sample. That was it.

Unless, of course, the amount of sugar still in her blood after an hour was outside the expected range. If that happened, then they'd suspect that her pancreas was not reliable under duress, and they'd start to adjust her diet and watch her blood sugar more closely. They would also do a full three-hour glucose-tolerance test, to be sure. The shorter version of the test occasionally gave falsely positive results, but it was easier than the full-blown version, and cheaper, and saved lots of patients from having to go through the complete testing.

It was worth it, Pupkin knew. It was worth a hundred tests, or five hundred, to identify the rare mother who might, in the latter part of pregnancy, unexpectedly develop diabetes. It was one thing when a diabetic woman wanted to have children and could plan for it. If she watched her blood sugar level with fanatic devotion, and if it was rock-steady at the time she conceived, then she could very likely avoid the bizarre deformities occasionally seen in the children of insulin-dependent diabetic women.

Diabetes during pregnancy constituted perhaps the highest risk of all to both the mother and the infant. Diabetic women often bore enormous babies, because the baby's pancreas functioned normally, allowing the baby to feast and grow huge on the mother's sugar-rich blood supply. The babies were completely normal in every respect, but were often too big to fit through the birth canal and had to be delivered by cesarean section. Sometimes diabetic women also developed high blood pressure, which doubled the problem and doubled the risk to mother and infant. If the high blood pressure turned into preeclampsia, sometimes the only way to save the mother's life was to terminate the pregnancy.

But worst of all, and the reason Laurie was getting the test, was that in the last weeks or days of pregnancy, the babies of diabetic women sometimes died, without warning or apparent reason, inside the uterus. Pupkin had seen cases where women were in labor, with everything progressing normally, when suddenly the needle on the fetal-heart monitor would begin to trace a flat line. Sometimes, on the way to the hospital, or during childbirth classes, or in the middle of the night, the mother would feel the infant give a final convulsive kick, and then there would be nothing.

Nobody knew why those babies died. Theories abounded, and Pupkin had heard most of them, but the truth was, nobody knew for sure. They knew from statistical studies that it only happened to a certain percentage of women and that in those women it seemed to happen again and again, but the numbers gave no answers. Obstetricians knew that, for such women, it was safest to induce labor, or perform a cesarean section, as soon as tests showed the baby's lungs were mature, and by that means they had made it safer for diabetic women to bear children, but no one could claim that the problem was solved or was even close to a solution.

Meanwhile, the first step was to identify people who were at risk. Pupkin twisted the cap off a small bottle and held it out. "Drink the whole thing," he said. Laurie accepted the bottle, which was labeled "Glucola." On Pupkin's advice she tossed it down in a single gulp, and then shuddered as the overwhelming sweetness began to assault her palate. She'd never tasted anything quite like it; the sweetness was so intense that it bordered on bitterness. She gulped once or twice, and her stomach felt slightly uneasy, but she gritted her teeth and handed back the bottle.

Pupkin made a sympathetic face. "It's pretty awful, isn't it?" he said. Laurie nodded.

After Pupkin finished the exam, Laurie sat and read magazines in the waiting room until the required hour had passed. Right on schedule, a nurse escorted her into a small room and drew a blood sample. They'd have results, she told Laurie, when she came for her next checkup.

The next checkup was only three weeks away. As she got nearer and nearer to term, the checkups would come at shorter and shorter intervals. Laurie felt a twinge of excitement. She was well past the halfway point now; soon—sooner than she wanted to think about—she'd have a baby. God, there were so many things to do!

The first thing she did, though, was phone Bill and instruct him where to meet her for lunch. Her pancreas must be working, she thought. Suddenly, she felt hungrier than she'd ever felt in her life.

A week later, Laurie returned, on a Thursday afternoon, to Dr. Bennett's office. Despite the late hour, a man in a three-piece suit and a woman with a small boy were still in the waiting room. Dr. Bennett was nowhere to be seen. Laurie gave her name to the receptionist and sat down.

She attempted to read an outdated copy of *People* magazine, but found herself studying the child opposite her. The boy looked to be about three. He was dressed in miniature designer jeans and was obviously restless. He crouched on the loveseat next to his mother and whined, endlessly, that he wanted to go home. His mother ignored him. The whining grew no louder, but neither did it diminish; it remained constant, high-pitched, nasal, petulant. After several minutes, Laurie began to wonder how the mother was able to tune it out. After several more minutes, she began to grow irritated. *Her* child, she vowed silently, would behave better in public.

A tall man with glasses and graying hair, wearing a dentist's smock, appeared at the doorway of the waiting room. That, Laurie thought, must be Big Mac. "Mr. Bivitch?" the dentist said, smiling. The man in the three-piece suit stood up and followed the dentist down the hallway. The child fell silent momentarily, watched the two men leave, then resumed his complaint.

Finally, Norma Bennett appeared, ushering a small girl, obviously the boy's older sister. "Here you are," Dr. Bennett said brightly to the mother. "All fixed up. What a nice little girl she is!" And what a rotten little brother she has, Laurie muttered to herself. Dr. Bennett exchanged pleasantries with the mother, then ushered her to the receptionist's desk, where the mother took out a checkbook. Dr. Bennett looked around, caught Laurie's eye, and with a jerk of her head motioned her toward the hallway, meanwhile bidding the mother and her two children goodbye.

Back in the treatment room, Dr. Bennett sat down heavily on a metal stool and shook with laughter. "What a family," she said. "The girl had a loose tooth, and rather than let it come out of its own accord, she brings the girl in here and pays me to take it out. The tooth was so loose I just lifted it out with my fingers. But the mother had her all worked up, so first, to calm her down, I told her a fairy tale, and then she told me about her secret uncle who comes to visit during the day when daddy's at work. Mercy! You think hairdressers hear it all, you should be a dentist!"

Laurie smiled. "There are no secrets when children are around," she said chuckling. "I'm going to have to get used to that in a couple of years."

"It's not too bad," Dr. Bennett said. "You don't lose your privacy forever, only for about twenty years."

"God, that sounds like a long time," Laurie said. "I sort of hate to have to admit that I'll be sixty when my baby turns twenty-one."

"Count your blessings. Imagine being sixty and having a teenager in the house. A boy, at that. Better late than never, I suppose, but I just hope I'll be up to it." As she talked, Dr. Bennett cleared the instrument table, then restocked it with fresh instruments and supplies. Laurie, who had sat down in the dentist's chair, watched a moment, then asked, "Do I need to have this tooth filled today?"

"Boy, am I glad you asked that," the dentist replied, "because the answer is no, and right now my feet hurt so bad that I want to cry. If you want to put it off, I won't complain at all."

"I want to put it off," Laurie said. "I feel like talking, and if I have a mouth full of novocaine, I'm not going to get a lot of talking done."

"Great," Dr. Bennett said. "Let's go out front so I can put my feet up."

The waiting room was empty. Dr. Bennett lowered herself onto one of the couches, kicked off her shoes, swung her feet up onto the couch and leaned back against the armrest. "Aaaaah," she sighed. "That's nice."

"Yeah," acknowledged Laurie, who had done the same thing on an adjacent couch. "It's a little extra weight, isn't it? But nice."

"So how did you celebrate when you got your results?" Dr. Bennett asked.

"Cautiously. I think I had two glasses of champagne. I actually got a little tipsy; that was the most I'd had to drink since I got pregnant."

Dr. Bennett laughed. "It's a real relief, isn't it? I don't know why everybody has to worry so much, but everybody does. Even when the odds are overwhelmingly in favor of everything being fine. You still worry."

"I like Trish's attitude about that," Laurie said. "Trish says it just means you care about your baby. That takes some of the pain out of worrying. Makes me feel like I'm doing something useful."

"Trish is great, didn't I tell you?" Dr. Bennett said. "Who else could talk me, a forty-five-year-old woman with two kids, into attending childbirth classes? *Childbirth classes*! Can you imagine?"

"When do you start the classes?" Laurie asked.

"I've already started," Dr. Bennett answered. "I'm at thirty-two weeks; that's when they like to start. The idea is that you finish the classes just in time to go into labor.

"Anyway, I've been to my first class," the dentist continued, "and Mac went with me. That's part of the idea, to get the husbands involved. Mac wasn't there for my first two deliveries; they didn't allow the fathers in the delivery room. This time, he gets to be there, and I think he's more thrilled than I am.

"Naturally, I went to this first class thinking there was nothing they could teach me, since I'd already been through it twice. Well, you wouldn't believe how much I learned. They never taught that sort of stuff in dental school!"

"They didn't teach it in law school, either," Laurie said. "I've got an obstetrics textbook, and I've learned a lot from that, but I still don't know what to expect."

"That's the beauty of classes," Dr. Bennett said. "I knew most of the physical or physiological things about childbirth when I had my girls," she said, "but I never put any thought into dealing with those things, or controlling them. I just let it happen to me, and I think I missed a lot because of that. The whole point of childbirth class is to teach you to participate."

"So what was the first one like?" Laurie asked.

"Oh, it was nice," Dr. Bennett said. "Remember consciousness-raising meetings back in the seventies? It was a lot like that. Mac got his consciousness raised quite a bit, and so did I. It's like anything else, the more you understand what you're doing, the better you can do it. This is going to be my last one, and I'm going to enjoy it. I don't want to miss a thing."

The phone on the receptionist's desk began to ring. With a groan of effort, Dr. Bennett swung around, hoisted herself up, and padded across the room in her stocking feet. "Dr. Bennett," she said into the phone.

She listened a moment, then said, crisply, "Yes. Bring him right over." She hung up and turned to Laurie, her face bleak. "It's a good thing we didn't do the filling today; we wouldn't have had any time to talk. That was a woman whose twelve-year-old just fell and knocked out two teeth. She's bringing him over now. Oh, God, my feet are gonna hurt!"

Painting the baby's room turned out to be a problem. Bill wanted to paint it light blue, and Laurie wanted a more neutral color, perhaps a light beige. They never got to the point of snarling over it, but they spent a good deal of time poring over color charts before they finally agreed on a pale yellow color called "flower petal," which Bill complained was a sissy name for paint but went along with.

Painting consumed one entire Saturday. Bill had bought some of the new pad-style paintbrushes and had jury-rigged a long pole with a clamp for the brush that was supposed to let him paint without using a ladder. It worked, after a fashion, but the pole had a tendency to bend under stress, and they finally worked out a system where Laurie would catch the brush end as Bill lowered it and would guide it to the pan of paint. Bill insisted that using a ladder would have been even more work.

In the end they had to use a ladder anyway, when it turned out that the pole simply would not stay steady enough to do the corners. By the time they were done, they both had paint all over them. Laurie had at least had the good sense to tie her hair in a handkerchief; Bill looked prematurely gray.

They showered together so Laurie could wash the paint out of Bill's hair, and ultimately she managed to do that, but not without a good bit of mutual fondling. After they finally dried each other off, they paraded naked to the bedroom, where they made love.

Laurie again brought up the question of intercourse when she went in for her twenty-nine-week checkup. Dr. Nagey was filling in that day, and he examined her abdomen, listened to the fetal heartbeat, let her listen to it, checked her blood pressure, and pronounced everything fine. In the consulting room, Laurie asked when she should stop having intercourse. Nagey made a face.

"There are honest differences of opinion about that," Nagey told her. "I always tell my patients that if it feels good, do it, and I mean just that; as long as it's not uncomfortable for you, it's okay, right up until you go into labor."

"I thought that could cause problems," Laurie said.

"A lot of people think that," Nagey replied, "and a lot of very good obstetricians still counsel their patients to abstain for the last four to six weeks. But that's a very conservative position. There have been studies on the subject, where one group abstained and another group didn't, and both groups had normal pregnancies, normal deliveries, and normal babies.

"If you were at risk for premature labor, we'd have told you to stop a long time ago. As long as you're sensible about it, you should have no problem."

"It's nice to get good news from a doctor," Laurie said. "Or have you been waiting till the last to tell me I have diabetes?"

"Diabetes?" Nagey looked puzzled.

"The glucose test," Laurie prompted.

"Oh, jeez, I forgot all about it," he replied, rummaging through the chart. "You must have done okay, or I would have heard something." He stopped, stared at a page briefly. "You sure did. You did fine."

[16]

Premature Labor

BY THE THIRTY-FIRST WEEK, Laurie had grown so large that neither she nor Bill could imagine her growing any larger. Walking had started to become a chore for her, and she was grateful that her work did not require her to sit directly in front of a desk. She had bought a plain wooden rocking chair for her office at the law firm, and rearranged things so that her telephone and dictating machine were within easy reach of it. She did most of her work rocking gently, with the chair tilted slightly to relieve the strain on her back. Once or twice she fell asleep in the chair. She seemed tired all the time now. It was not the sickly fatigue she'd felt early in the pregnancy; she was simply bone-tired, exhausted, and no amount of rest seemed to revive her.

She continued to take walks, but she had long since abandoned tennis. She wanted to exercise more, but the strength wasn't there, and self-discipline could drive her only so far. Lately, even the walks had become shorter and shorter. Some days, she didn't walk at all.

Bill, sympathetic as ever, always walked with her, always encouraged her to walk as far as she could, but never pushed it when she wanted to quit. Bill claimed to enjoy the walks, which he described as his opportunity to strut alongside his pregnant bride. Laurie had scoffed when he'd first said it, but the thought had stayed with her, and she'd begun to notice how much differently the world seemed to treat her. Strangers smiled and greeted her on the street; she hardly ever opened a door herself anymore. People cleared space for her on elevators and invited her to go ahead of them in checkout lines. Even the law firm's senior partner, who had complained bitterly about the damage Laurie's pregnancy would cause to the firm's schedule, was downright courtly whenever he encountered her in the hallways of the office, and once when he'd passed her on the street, he'd actually tipped his hat.

The pregnancy had indeed changed her life, she reflected, just as it had changed the lives of so many of their friends years before. Laurie had lunch with one of her old college friends who now had two teenage sons and a second husband. The woman reminisced about her own pregnancies, which had been uneventful, except that near the end her ankles had become so badly swollen she could hardly walk. Both sons had been delivered under anesthesia; she didn't remember a lot about either time, she said. Then the conversation turned to the perils of child-rearing.

The Walkers, Jim and Robbie, were the only couple with whom Laurie and Bill had maintained contact over the years. The Walkers were also childless, for much the same reasons as Laurie and Bill: Both had careers. They had invited Laurie and Bill for dinner not long after Laurie had learned she was pregnant, and had seemed genuinely thrilled when Laurie made her announcement. More recently, Laurie and Bill had invited them over, and during dinner, Robbie asked casually how the pregnancy was going. Laurie launched into a lengthy recitation of all the trials and tribulations of pregnancy, but finally caught herself.

"Jeez, I sound like all the others, don't I?" she said.

Robbie grinned, said nothing.

"I guess it does sort of dominate your life," Laurie went on. "I still practice law, and I still do all the things I always did, but now my priorities are all rearranged."

"Oh, it'll get worse," Robbie said cheerfully. "Just wait till the baby's born."

"Yeah," Laurie mused. "Next time you see me I'll be up to my elbows in diapers and Dr. Spock."

"And now you know why I'm going to let you have all the babies for both of us," Robbie said.

There goes the old peer group, Laurie reflected, once again, as the conversation moved on to other topics.

She'd even noticed a change in the demeanor of the judges

before whom she practiced. Laurie had been flattered, but later furious when a panel of three appellate judges had treated her with uncommon politeness, wished her a successful pregnancy, and then ruled against her.

The case where being pregnant had clearly been a bonus was the nagging child-custody case that had turned into a paternity suit. Laurie had done some checking and discovered that the same division of human genetics that had done her amniocentesis could also do a series of blood assays, which, taken together, could determine with great accuracy whether people were related.

The two girls and their father dutifully gave blood samples. The man who was claiming to be the real father refused. At a preliminary hearing, Laurie apologetically asked the judge if she might be permitted to enter a last-minute motion. "I've been running behind schedule," she said, glancing meaningfully at her middle.

"Counselor, the Court is aware that you're on a schedule of your own, and I think we can certainly accommodate that," the judge replied. The defense attorney nodded warily. He could have objected, but it would have been, well, ungentlemanly.

As Laurie then read aloud her motion to dismiss based on the blood-test results and the putative father's refusal, she handed the judge and defense attorney copies of the lab reports. Then the defense attorney, red-faced and sputtering, objected loudly and at length, but it was too late. The test results showed a probability of greater than ninety percent that Laurie's client was the girls' natural father. The judge let the defense attorney storm and bluster awhile, then cut him off.

"Counsel, in the interest of conserving the court's time, I'm going to postpone this case indefinitely, until you can bring me some equally convincing evidence that your client's claim isn't frivolous. Adjourned."

The defense attorney and his clients glared at Laurie as she left the courtroom. She smiled sweetly and waved to them. The case should have gone to trial: Technically, the judge's ruling was incorrect and, if challenged, could be easily overturned. But now that they knew what sort of evidence Laurie had available, she doubted they'd press the matter. She grinned to herself. She hadn't had this much fun since she was a prosecutor. Then, in the next instant, she grimaced and rubbed her back. It seemed that her back was sore all the time lately. Another symptom of pregnancy, no doubt. It was a good thing she didn't have to spend too much time in court. You did a lot of standing up and sitting down in courtrooms, and that was something Laurie found increasingly difficult to do.

Happily, Laurie's most lucrative job lately was reading. Her expertise in the antitrust field had made her an overnight success, and she'd been kept busy consulting with other members of the firm, reading long, detailed, complex descriptions of existing or contemplated business maneuvers and dispensing opinions on whether or not one business deal or another would violate antitrust laws. It was the sort of thing that could usually be done from a rocking chair.

At home, Bill continued to pamper her as much as she would allow, which was not a lot, but still more than she was used to. They usually ate early, went for their walks before dark, and spent quiet evenings at home. It had become uncomfortable for Laurie to sit for a long time in theater seats; since her back hurt all the time, sometimes she let Bill put a heating pad in the recliner that she sat in at home.

The evening snack had become a ritual. Some nights they had delicatessen-style cold-cut sandwiches, other times toasted bagels with cream cheese, or fruit and cheese with crackers, and an occasional glass of wine. Laurie, who had long been accustomed to a regular happy hour, now sipped her wine gingerly, mindful of what she'd read about fetal alcohol syndrome.

They still made love occasionally, having found a position that was comfortable for both of them. Afterward, Bill liked to lie diagonally across the huge bed, with his head, and usually one hand, resting lightly against Laurie's middle as though it were a fragile pillow. That was how, on the fifth day of the thirty-first week, a Thursday night, Bill was the first to notice something odd.

"You know, this is hard as a rock tonight," he complained, brushing his ear lightly against the side of her abdomen. "Are you doing that on purpose?"

"Doing what?" Laurie asked, putting her hands on either side of her navel. "You're right," she said. "I hadn't even noticed. It doesn't hurt. I wonder—God, maybe I'm in labor."

"Labor, hell," Bill replied, raising himself on an elbow and making a show of buffing his nails on his chest. "You probably just got too excited. I can't help it that I'm so good."

"No, this is serious," Laurie said. "Feel. It's really tight, all over, and especially on top. Something's wrong. I think I'm having a contraction."

"You thought you had toxemia, too. And diabetes, and cervical cancer, and . . . " Bill ticked off diseases on his fingers. "Face it, you're a hypochondriac."

"It's relaxing now," Laurie reported. "Now feel." She guided Bill's hand back. "Feel the difference? It was really tight before."

Bill pulled himself up parallel to Laurie, slipped an arm under her head, and settled into their traditional cuddling position. She snuggled closer. "Okay," he said, "you had a contraction. You yourself told me about false labor. You read it to me out of that goddam book of yours, the Nixon's Claxons contractions . . . "

"Braxton-Hicks contractions," Laurie corrected, giggling.

" . . . whatever the hell they are, and that's what you probably just had one of, since you don't like my theory about delayed orgasm."

"Oh, shut up and hug," Laurie hissed. After that, they lay quiet for a long time. They were almost asleep when the next contraction started.

Bill's hand was still resting on her abdomen, and he felt it begin to tighten. "Oh, shit," he said. "Oh, shit. That's not an orgasm, is it?"

Laurie wasn't listening. She already had the bedside lamp on and was reaching for the telephone.

Four hours into her shift, the delivery-room nurse had decided it was going to be a rotten night. She had arrived just in time to help the chief resident deliver a fifteen-year-old girl who lived in one of the ghettos to the west of the hospital complex and who, twenty weeks into her first pregnancy, had gone into labor. She had showed up, alone and frightened, in the emergency room, her shoes sopping wet. The ER staff had put her into a wheelchair and rushed her upstairs, where the chief resident, a senior resident, and a second-year resident had worked heroically for several hours to stop the labor, but to no avail. At eleven minutes after ten, the woman had delivered a five-inch, twelve-ounce fetus, which made several convulsive movements with its arms before it died.

The nurse had dutifully removed the fetus, wrapped in a towel, to the newborn room, where she'd weighed it, measured its length, and somberly recorded the pertinent facts in the official delivery-room log book. The newborn room was usually a happier place, resounding with the furious protests of babies during their first bath or the head-to-toe exam that preceded it. Right now the place was like a morgue, quiet and sepulchral. It gave her the creeps, and she was glad to get out. The fetus lay, covered, in a stainless-steel tray, awaiting a trip to the pathology department for autopsy.

She had returned to the nurses' station in time to answer a phone call from a woman who was thirty-nine weeks pregnant and upset because her legs hurt and her ankles were swollen. She had spoken with the woman several times before, and had also spoken with the woman's doctor before. The nurse assured the woman, one more time, that it would all be over soon and ended the conversation as politely, but as rapidly, as she could. Another line was ringing.

This time it was the charge nurse from the patient ward just down the hall. A patient who'd been admitted that morning after her membranes ruptured had now begun to have regular contractions and should be moved to one of the labor rooms. There was a note of urgency in the charge nurse's voice. "She's a screamer," the nurse said, "and she's upsetting everybody else."

The delivery-room nurse hung up the phone with a sigh. Screamers were not uncommon, nor were they particularly difficult or unpleasant patients; they were simply people with low pain thresholds, people who had been taught from infancy that screams of pain brought love. Their pain was, doubtless, real; but it was somehow amplified almost beyond endurance. Oddly—or perhaps not so oddly—screamers often refused anesthesia. The delivery-room nurse dispatched two other nurses to fetch the screamer.

The chief resident, who had delivered the premature fetus, showed up at the nurses' station looking grim. University Hospital, a third-level care center, saw more than its share of bad pregnancies, but each loss was a fresh sadness, a shared grieving. But it was especially wrenching for this particular chief resident, who was herself twenty-three weeks pregnant. The chief resident had the advantage of being twenty-seven years old instead of fifteen, and had the further advantage of good diet, good medical advice, good sense, and a good husband, but it was impossible for her not to identify with the girl, and her face was bleak. "She wants to see it," she said. The nurse nodded quietly, and the two women walked back to the newborn room.

They took what seemed like a very long time arranging the fetus, wrapping it in a white cotton cloth, much the way they'd have swathed a live newborn, with only the face showing. They walked back to the delivery room, and the nurse, carrying the fetus, hung back out of sight behind the bedside curtain while the chief resident consulted with the two junior residents, speaking in the medical argot that physicians use to conceal their bedside discussions from the patients being discussed. The girl had lost less than one unit of blood, the resident said, and transfusion did not seem necessary. They'd sent a fresh blood sample to the lab to be sure. The placenta had come out intact and without problems, and the woman seemed to be doing fine, including "depressed affect," which is a doctor's clinical description of profound sorrow, and which would have been remarkable only if it had been absent.

The nurse could hear the change in the chief resident's voice, from clinical to bedside, and she heard the patient mumble acknowledgments. "Do you want to see your baby now?" the chief resident asked. The nurse couldn't hear a reply, but after a moment the chief resident said, softly, "Okay." The nurse walked around to the side of the bed, cradling the dead fetus as though it were her own, stood close to the bedside, and held the bundle out toward the mother, forearm supporting the body, just like always.

The girl was not pretty—she was overweight, her skin was dark and slightly mottled, her hair was matted and greasy, and her teeth were misshapen and stained—but in her dark eyes was a pain that is universal. She did not take the baby in her hands, but only stared at it for a long time. Then she lifted one hand and touched the baby's face lightly with a grimy finger. The tears began to well up in the girl's eyes, and she turned her head away. The nurse stepped back from the bed and, at a nod from the chief resident, carried the tiny corpse back to the newborn room. As she walked down the hallway, the double doors at the far end swung open and a gurney, pushed by two nurses, rolled through. As it did, the patient on the gurney announced her presence with a series of gasps culminating in a gargling, teeth-clenched scream. It was going to be a very long night.

From the newborn room, she walked back to the nurses' station and sat down heavily on a stool. It was eleven-thirty. When the telephone rang, her arm shot out automatically, but unenthusiastically. "Delivery room," she answered.

It was Dr. Crenshaw. He spoke quietly, clearly, briefly. He had a private patient, Laura Edwards, who'd had two contractions within twenty minutes after having intercourse. She was thirty-one weeks pregnant. She was on her way downtown right now. The nurse should alert the residents, pull Edwards's chart, and, just to be safe, make sure there was a bed available in the intensive-care nursery.

"We'll be ready," she replied.

The labor-and-delivery suite at the University of Maryland

Hospital was one of the most modern and sophisticated obstetric wards in Baltimore when it was built, in the early 1950s. Almost thirty-five years later it was still serviceable, but like a thirty-five-year-old car, or a thirty-five-year-old dress, it was hopelessly out of date. The delivery suite was cold and antiseptic, gloomy, and inhospitable, a relic of a time when childbirth was regarded as an ailment, a disease to be treated, a trauma to be repaired.

The history of that delivery suite was a history of steady decline in the hospital's obstetrics program or, more charitably, an unwillingness to keep pace with the expectations of an increasingly consumerist generation of mothers. By the late 1970s, the university's obstetric clientele was largely limited to public-assistance patients from the surrounding ghettos.

When, in 1979, the University of Maryland's medical school and hospital were trying to woo Carlyle Crenshaw away from Duke to rebuild the department of obstetrics and gynecology at Maryland, one of the first things they had to do was promise him a new labor-and-delivery suite. The existing one, Crenshaw said bluntly, was hopelessly out of date, inadequate for the needs of modern obstetric practice, an affront to the patients he would try to attract. It was, or ought to be, an embarrassment to the hospital.

As with any state institution the work began slowly, with endless budget hearings, planning sessions, design meetings, and consultations with every minor functionary or ad hoc committee that might lay a territorial claim to some trivial part of the process and which, if ignored, would somehow manage to block progress until protocol was satisfied. Crenshaw had chafed and bristled, blustered and bullied, and occasionally pleaded. Finally, four years later, construction had begun on the new delivery suite, one floor above the present one. Ironically, only a few months after the work started, the state created a private nonprofit corporation to run University Hospital, thus freeing it from much of the labyrinthine bureaucracy that state institutions are burdened with.

Now the hospital's managers answered to a board of directors, and as Crenshaw's department continued its renovation program, that very short chain of command could make things happen more easily and more quickly. Soon there would be no more four-patient rooms; soon every room would have its own bathroom. Not long after that, there would be a sophisticated outpatient clinic, designed to allow patients to avoid the expense and inconvenience of hospitalization whenever possible. Then, at last, the hospital's physical facilities would match the caliber of the obstetrics-and-gynecology staff Crenshaw had assembled, and patients would no longer have to sacrifice comfort and dignity to be cared for by Crenshaw's team of experts.

The capstone of that renovation plan would be the new labor-and-delivery suite, and it would be opening soon, in only a few more weeks. The new suite would reflect, as its predecessor thirty-five years before had reflected, not only the present state of medical and obstetrical art, but also the attitudes and philosophies of the physicians and their patients. There would be birthing rooms, with comfortable furniture and soft lighting to replace the stainless steel and polished tile of the old delivery rooms. There would be birthing beds, designed for the mother's comfort as much as for the doctor's convenience. All the high technology, the monitors, the tools, the myriad supplies, would be seconds away in case they were needed, but they would be out of sight, unobtrusive. The new suite would combine the comfort and intimacy of home birth with the security of having expert medical care instantly available if something went wrong.

But the labor-and-delivery suite that greeted Laurie and Bill at eleven fifty-one that night was the 1950s version, and as she walked down the hallway, Laurie entertained serious doubts about her choice of hospitals.

To get to the delivery suite at all, it was necessary to walk from the sixth floor elevator lobby of the north hospital building into the older south building, down a series of hallways that led back past offices and consultation rooms, through double doors, and into a hallway lined with semiprivate hospital rooms. The hallway ended at the old building's octagonal rotunda and the nurses' station in the center of it. A hand-painted sign on yellow posterboard pointed down another hallway to the delivery rooms, and that one seemed even older and more dimly lit than the one before it. There were more semiprivate rooms along the hallway.

A metal door blocked the way to the delivery suite itself, and there were large red signs on it. One announced that beyond those doors lay the delivery room. The second warned the unauthorized to stay out, while the third sign invited Laurie to ring the bell twice if she was a patient, once if a visitor. She located the push button, rang twice, and waited. Shortly, a nurse wearing a green scrub suit opened the door. From somewhere behind the nurse an agonized "Aaaarrrgh!" echoed out of one of the rooms and down the hallway.

"I'm Mrs. Edwards," Laurie said quietly.

Less than two minutes later, Laurie was supine on the examining table in the first room past the doorway. The nurse had showed her to a small bathroom off the examining room and handed her a hospital gown and a paper bag. Laurie put her clothes in the bag, put on the hospital gown, and emerged into the examining room, where the nurse helped her onto the table. Functionally, the room was much like the examining rooms in Crenshaw's private offices, but this one had tile walls, two examining tables, and a bewildering array of cabinets, shelves, carts, trays, lights, monitors, and supply packages. Everywhere Laurie looked, stainless steel and sterile green cloth greeted her. She glanced at the foot of the other examining table; sure enough, they even had the little rolling stainless-steel trashcans.

A resident in a scrub suit introduced himself to Laurie and said he'd spoken to Dr. Crenshaw at home. "I'll stay in touch with him," the resident said, "and he'll come downtown if necessary. First, we need to find out what's happening."

While the nurse checked her blood pressure and pulse, the resident shot a rapid-fire string of questions at Laurie and, sensing the man's urgency, she answered them rapidly. Yes, she was still having contractions, and they were becoming more frequent. No, she hadn't timed them. Membranes? Ruptured? Oh. No. No, her water hadn't broken. Yes, she'd found a spot of blood just now when she undressed.

"Get an IV ready, will you?" the resident said to the nurse, then, to Laurie, "Let me check your cervix and see if it's started to dilate."

He helped Laurie fit her legs into the stirrups, quickly pulled on an examining glove, and probed the back of her vagina for several seconds. The tip of the cervix had begun to dilate, but it wouldn't quite accept the resident's fingertip. However, as the resident moved his fingers along the length of the cervix, he could feel that it had begun to efface, to thin out. Now there was no question. Laurie was in labor.

"We'll need a CBC and a sterile specimen," the resident told the nurse as he pulled off the examining glove. "I've got to use the phone." He left.

"Stay up in the stirrups, hon," the nurse advised Laurie. "I've got to get a sterile urine sample from you, but I've got to do the bloods and the IV first. This'll just take a second."

Working quickly, the nurse drew two small vials of blood from Laurie's left arm. A bag of intravenous fluid was already hanging on a pole beside the bed, and as soon as the nurse laid the vials of blood aside, she opened a sterile plastic package, withdrew an IV needle and tube, and expertly inserted it in a vein in the crook of Laurie's left arm. She hooked it to the bag of fluid and opened a valve all the way, and the sterile water, laced with dissolved salt and sugar, flowed into Laurie's bloodstream.

Another series of gasping screams echoed down the hallway, "Oh! . . . oh! Oh! OH! . . . OH! . . . AH! . . . AAAAH! . . . AAAAARGH!" but the nurse appeared not to notice.

"Jesus," Laurie said. "What's wrong with that woman?"

"Nothing," the nurse replied. "Labor."

"You mean that's normal?"

"For her it is. This is her third child."

"She sounds like she's dying. Can't you give her something for the pain?"

"We could give her lots of things," the nurse replied, "but she doesn't want any of them."

"Oh," Laurie said. "I hope she has her baby soon."

"So do we, hon, so do we," said the nurse.

While they talked, she broke open another sterile package containing gauze pads, stainless-steel forceps to hold them, antiseptic, a sterile plastic container, and a Foley catheter. With a brief word of explanation to Laurie, the nurse pulled on sterile gloves, soaked a gauze pad in dark-brown antiseptic, and began to swab Laurie's labia. Urine in the bladder is sterile, but all sorts of bacteria live near the tip of the urethra, and obtaining a urine sample under sterile conditions is yet another of the undignified experiences incident to womanhood.

Still holding the labia open with her left hand, the nurse picked up the small catheter, dipped the tip of it in a small container of sterile lubricant, placed the tip against the opening of the urethra, and pushed gently. Deftly, the nurse pushed the catheter farther, farther, farther inside until suddenly the clear plastic tube turned yellow and urine began to fill the plastic specimen container. The nurse waited a moment, then withdrew the catheter. Perfect.

The urine specimen would go immediately to the laboratory, where a technician would put it in a centrifuge, spin it for a few minutes at high speed, and see what collected at the bottom. The report would be available within half an hour.

The resident reported to Crenshaw that Laurie's cervix was barely dilated, but that it was substantially effaced, fifty percent, perhaps a little more. She was having contractions about every six minutes now. The resident had already started giving her fluids, and was sending blood and urine samples to the lab. Crenshaw murmured his approval, then added, "If she doesn't respond to the fluids fairly rapidly, start her on Ritodrine and let me know. If that doesn't work, I'll come down and deliver her. Did you find out if there were any beds in the nursery?"

"Yes, sir," the resident said. "They're full. They said they don't have any more room."

There was a long silence at the other end of the phone. Both Crenshaw and the resident knew what that meant. At thirty-one weeks, a baby had a ninety-plus percent chance of surviving, in an intensive-care nursery. Without the intensive-care nursery, the chance of survival was zero.

Finally, Crenshaw sighed. "I'll talk to them. You go try to get her stopped."

[17]
Contractions and Ritodrine

CRENSHAW hung up the phone and dialed Trish Payne's number. One of Trish's jobs was to coordinate patient transfers to the four intensive-care nurseries in Baltimore. His frown intensified as he listened to Trish explain that all the beds in the city had been full for two days and none of the hospitals anticipated a discharge for at least another two days. She had been refusing transfers from all over the state, she said. Crenshaw sighed, thanked her, broke the connection, and dialed the intensive-care nursery at University Hospital.

It was a familiar crisis, but it was a fresh frustration every time it happened, a fresh lesson in the hypocrisy and ignorance of which government was ever capable: The same government that poured its resources into "Baby Doe" regulations was daily responsible for the deaths of dozens of premature infants.

Medicaid—medical assistance for the poor—programs are operated by individual states, but they are heavily funded by the federal government. As federal funds have begun to diminish, Medicaid programs nationwide have cut back on the services they pay for. One of the obvious solutions, and one that has been adopted in many states, has been to limit the number of days a public-assistance patient may be hospitalized. In Maryland, the limit was twenty days.

The large hospitals, like the University of Maryland Hospital, protested vehemently: Maryland's world-famous Shock-Trauma Center was located at University Hospital, and very few of their Medicaid patients could be discharged in only twenty days; the average stay of a premature baby was something in excess of two months. If Medicaid funding were cut off after twenty days, UMH—and the other hospitals that run similar programs—would lose so much money that they would simply have to discontinue the programs. Or refuse to admit Medicaid patients.

The government gave in to the pressure and granted a waiver to trauma centers and intensive-care nurseries. And in doing so, it set up the macabre irony that now faced Carlyle Crenshaw—or, more correctly, that now faced Laura and Bill Edwards and their unborn baby. Premature infants need intensive, high-technology life support until they reach the level of maturity found at about thirty-four weeks of gestation. For about a month after that, the infants require close monitoring in a hospital setting, but the crisis is over. They no longer need the sophisticated, twenty-four-hour service of the intensive-care nursery.

But if they're not in the nursery, Medicaid won't pay for them. This has left many of the nation's intensive-care nurseries jammed with Medicaid babies who don't belong there but have nowhere else to go. University Hospital alone could admit another ten premature babies a month if they could weed out the ones who don't belong there.

Ironically, the babies who die are the ones born to the middle-class suburban and small-town families whose community hospitals do not deliver enough premature babies to justify their own intensive-care nurseries. It is the rare ironic case where Reagan Administration policies have led to discrimination in *favor* of the poor.

The resident silently cursed the evils of bureaucracy as he walked back to the admitting room. He saw Bill sitting on a plastic chair outside the room, stopped, and introduced himself. "She's having premature labor," the resident said, "but at this stage we can sometimes stop it. I'm going to talk to your wife now. You're welcome to come in, too."

Bill stood up and walked into the examining room with him. Laurie was still lying on the table, no longer in the stirrups. "You're definitely having premature labor," the resident told Laurie, "and we don't know why. We're giving you intravenous fluids right now, and very often that alone will stop the labor.

"Right now we want to move you to a room across the hall

where we can use a monitor to keep track of how the baby's doing and also to tell us when you have a contraction. If we don't get you stopped, or substantially slowed down within half an hour or so, there are some other things we can try."

"What happens if I have the baby tonight?" Laurie asked.

"At thirty-one weeks, he'll have a ninety-five-plus percent chance of survival," the resident replied, praying silently that Crenshaw would be able to twist enough arms to free up a bed, "and he'll spend two very long, very frustrating months in the intensive-care nursery." If we can get a bed, the resident added to himself.

The resident and Bill helped Laurie down from the examining table and the nurse, pushing the wheeled IV pole, followed Laurie, as she clutched the hospital gown behind her and crossed the hallway to a labor room with a single bed next to a large electronic device. As soon as Laurie was arranged in the bed, the nurse began placing sensors on her abdomen. The monitor gave off a slushy, liquid sound that Laurie now recognized as the Doppler heartbeat monitor. The nurse pressed a button, and a strip of paper, showing the tracing of the fetal heart rate, began to advance slowly from the machine.

Lying on her back, Laurie couldn't see the monitor; but she could feel the contractions, and while they didn't get any worse or any more rapid, neither did they diminish. Bill sat by the bed. They tried to talk about other things, but without success, and there was little they could say about the night's events, so they were soon silent. Laurie's mood was bleak. She'd never felt so completely helpless.

The resident came in every few minutes, spoke to Laurie, checked the lengthening strip of paper, and left. Finally, when the first IV bag was nearly empty, the resident and the nurse walked in and stood by the bed. The contractions were not diminishing, the resident explained, and if they continued much longer, Laurie would have a baby tonight. That would be a real problem, the resident said, since the intensive-care nursery was terribly crowded at the moment and there was some question as to where the baby would go. They would find a bed somehow if they had to, the resident promised, but obviously, he added, the baby would be better off if he could spend the next two months inside Laurie, where he belonged. Toward that end, he told Laurie and Bill, he was recommending that they start treating her with a drug called Ritodrine.

For a woman in premature labor, Ritodrine can be a miracle drug and, properly used, it often is. But it is a very dangerous drug, with a number of serious side effects. The most common one is rapid heartbeat and tension, a jittery feeling that won't go away. But Ritodrine also causes blood sugar levels to go up and blood potassium levels to go down. The distance between systolic and diastolic blood pressure widens, and there is a remote chance that the mother will develop congestive heart failure. Those complications can usually be avoided by calibrating the dose carefully, but the therapy is not without risk, the resident said, and they would not use it unless Laurie and Bill, understanding those risks, agreed that it was a good idea.

Laurie and Bill agreed.

Within minutes a second IV pole was standing beside Laurie's bed. This one had a small blue electronic box attached to it, and the Ritodrine-laced saline solution flowed through a tiny vial built into the side of the blue box before exiting into the tube that led to Laurie's left arm. The blue box was an automatic measuring device that metered precisely the amount of Ritodrine dispensed. Too much and Laurie would have severe side effects; too little and she'd have a baby. To reach the middle ground they'd have to titrate.

Titration, as every high school student learns in chemistry class, is the process of adding a chemical to a solution, drop by drop, until the desired result is obtained. Chemistry teachers make it a game, adding random quantities of acid to water, then adding an indicator to turn it pink. When the acid is completely neutralized, the liquid suddenly turns clear. The object is to add just that amount and no more. Add too much alkali to the solution and it turns blue, and you lose.

Titrating Laurie was the same sort of project, but do it wrong and you might lose Laurie. Or her baby. Or both. So for the first ten minutes, Laurie received a Ritodrine dose of 100 micrograms—millionths of a gram—per minute, the smallest dose ever reported to have stopped premature labor. The resident didn't really expect that dose to work, but he had to start somewhere.

They would have to stop somewhere, too. The highest dose ever safely administered was 350 micrograms per minute, and at that level the side effects could be severe, so severe that there was a second critical measurement: Laurie's pulse rate. If it got above one hundred forty, the Ritodrine dose would have to be reduced, and Laurie would probably have her baby.

The resident and the nurse bustled in and out of the labor room incessantly. One or the other was almost always there, constantly checking Laurie's pulse, examining the strip of paper emerging from the fetal monitor for any signs that the baby was in distress and, at the same time, calculating the length of time between contractions. The monitor strip usually showed a row of sharp, low, closely spaced spikes representing the baby's heartbeat. During a contraction, the line would swing slowly up and down, marking the spot. The paper itself was calibrated in minutes.

Laurie's contractions were still six minutes apart. Her pulse was one hundred. She had a contraction just after the Ritodrine was started, and six minutes later she had another one. Pulse one hundred, steady.

Two minutes later, the nurse raised the Ritodrine dose to 150 micrograms per minute. Four minutes later, Laurie had a contraction. Pulse one hundred five. Six minutes more, and she had another one.

The nurse raised the dose to 200 micrograms. Laurie's pulse rate was now one hundred fifteen. Six minutes, and Laurie had a contraction. The nurse waited four more minutes, raised the dose to 250.

Two minutes later the nurse, watching the monitor, held a hand on Laurie's abdomen, waiting for the contraction, watching the pulse, one hundred twenty, steady, waiting . . . waiting . . . six and a half . . . one-twenty and steady . . . waiting . . . seven . . . waiting . . . seven and a half . . .

The contraction came eight minutes after the last one, and the nurse gave a little whoop of joy. Good medical practice dictated that it was far too early to reassure Laurie and Bill, but there was no hiding the nurse's glee. "No promises," she told them, "but I think it's going to work." She left the Ritodrine steady at 250 micrograms, waited. Six minutes, seven, eight . . . eight and a half, nine, nine and a half . . . and another contraction. The pulse remained steady at one hundred twenty. The nurse began humming softly to herself.

The resident walked in, looking pleased. He'd just spoken to the lab, he told Laurie and Bill, and the good news was that she had a urinary infection.

"That's good news?" Laurie asked.

"It sure is," the resident replied. "That's probably what caused you to start contracting. I just hope you're not allergic to penicillin."

A few minutes later, the nurse added a third bag of fluid to the tangle of intravenous equipment hanging beside Laurie's bed. This one contained ampicillin, a synthetic form of penicillin, mixed with the ever-present sterile saline. The Ritodrine continued at 250 micrograms per minute.

The next contraction occurred at twelve minutes; then seventeen; then twenty-one. Then the contractions stopped.

[18]

In the Hospital

BILL insisted on staying at Laurie's bedside that night despite Laurie's protests. Anywhere else in the hospital, the campus police, who enforce visiting hours very strictly, would have thrown Bill out. In the labor and delivery suite, visiting hours are twenty-four hours a day.

Laurie stayed in the labor room for nine more hours. Nurses checked her pulse and blood pressure every fifteen minutes and kept close track of what she drank and what she excreted. Several times during the night, nurses drew fresh blood samples to send to the lab.

When, after six hours, she'd had no further contractions, the resident and the nurse began reducing the dosage of Ritodrine by 50 micrograms every half hour, until she was back to the original dosage of 100 micrograms per minute. The paper strip, now several yards long, emerged slowly from the machine, showing a steady, healthy fetal heart rate and no contractions. After a half hour, they allowed her to stand up, experimentally, for a few minutes. Still no contractions.

The nurse came in with a pill, handed it to Laurie. "This is more Ritodrine," she explained. "You can start taking it orally now, and we'll discontinue the IV in about another hour."

Laurie took the pill, and the nurse left. A moment later, Dr. Crenshaw walked in. "Good morning," he said cheerily. "And congratulations."

"Congratulations?" Laurie said. "We almost screwed things up. Literally."

Crenshaw shook his head. "There's probably no amount of reassurance that will convince you, but I don't think this had anything to do with having intercourse. You have a bladder infection, and that is almost surely the cause. I think it was a coincidence that you noticed the contractions right after intercourse. And I have to add that if you hadn't noticed them when you did, we'd probably have a baby on our hands this morning, and I wouldn't have gotten any sleep. So thank you for paying attention."

"Thank him," Laurie said, nodding her head toward the corner, where Bill was sound asleep in a chair. "He spotted it first."

Crenshaw grinned. "Thank you both for helping," he said. "In gratitude, I'll try to let you get some sleep soon. I've reserved a private room for you, and as soon as we discontinue the intravenous Ritodrine, we'll move you down there. You'll be taking a Ritodrine tablet every four hours, but we'll leave the other IV in for a while yet. If everything goes well, we might send you home tomorrow."

"I'll be back to normal that soon?" Laurie asked.

"Not back to normal, no. We'll want you to stay in bed for the next couple of weeks. Don't do any more walking than you have to, and no physical exertion, of course. No intercourse. We don't want to take any chances at all."

"How likely is this to happen again?" she asked.

"If you take the Ritodrine religiously, not very. You responded to it very quickly last night, and that's an encouraging sign. We know that works now, so we'll simply keep you on Ritodrine until it doesn't matter whether or not you go into labor. Before then, we'll want to check you every couple of days, and if you get through the next week or two with no more problems, then you can go back to work part time."

"What about classes?" Laurie demanded. "My classes start next week."

"I'll talk to Trish," Crenshaw said. "Let's see how you look next week."

The private room Laurie was put into was sheerest luxury. It was one of a scant half-dozen rooms that had already been renovated, and the room was bright, modern, compact, private, and had its own bathroom. They moved Laurie into the room on a gurney, helped her onto the bed, arranged all her IVs and then, mercifully, left her alone for two hours, while she got the first sleep she'd had in twenty-four hours. They woke her at eleven for her Ritodrine pill, and at eleven-thirty an orderly brought her a lunch tray. The food was typically gray-looking institutional food, but Laurie wolfed it down and wished for more. She'd been too tired before to notice how hungry she was.

In the afternoon, she paid to have the television hooked up and watched two soap operas before she dozed off. At three o'clock a nurse woke her and gave her a Ritodrine tablet. At four-thirty they fed her again. At five-thirty Bill showed up with flowers in his hand and bags under his eyes, and Laurie harangued him until he agreed to go home and get a good night's sleep.

At seven o'clock, she got a Ritodrine pill. At eight, a nurse removed the last IV from Laurie's arm. At eleven, they gave her the Ritodrine pill and an antibiotic. Laurie fell asleep during the late news. At three o'clock, the nurse woke her for another pill.

The next morning Dr. Nagey stopped in early, chatted awhile, examined Laurie's cervix, pronounced it improved, and promised that if she continued to improve, she could go home the following day. A few minutes after he left, Trish Payne walked in.

"Some people," she began, "will do anything to get out of going to classes."

"I was just complaining about that myself," Laurie said wryly. "It's all Bill's fault, you know."

"That's the spirit," Trish said. "Seriously, I looked through your chart, and I wanted to make sure they'd told you that the cause was apparently a bladder infection and not . . . anything else."

"You mean screwing," Laurie said bluntly.

"Right," said Trish. "Everybody believes that was a lucky coincidence. So do I."

"Lucky?"

"Sure. What if you'd gone to sleep instead? The chart said you never complained of any pain. You might not have noticed until you were too far gone for us to stop you. If it was going to happen, you couldn't have picked a better time for it to happen.''

"Okay," Laurie said, unconvinced.

"The important thing," Trish went on, "is that you and your husband don't get caught up in some guilt trip now and give up sex because it might be bad for the baby.''

"Dr. Crenshaw already told me to give up sex," Laurie said.

"The only reason for that is because physiologically you're still sort of in labor right now. The Ritodrine has stopped the contractions, but your cervix is still effaced, and just a tiny bit dilated. If you had intercourse right now, you could break your membranes, and then there'd be no way we'd get you to term. The reason they want you to lie down for the next couple of weeks is to take the pressure off your cervix, give it a chance to firm up a little.''

"Okay, okay," Laurie said. "I'll be good. More important, can I go to classes?''

"I'd hate for you to miss the first class," Trish said. "I'll do some lobbying with Dr. Crenshaw. Meanwhile, stay in bed for as much of this next week as you can. We'll figure something out.''

Twelve hours later, Trish showed up again. Laurie switched off the television. "You do work long hours," she said to Trish.

"Oh, I've been home. I came back for a special occasion. I thought you'd like to know. Norma Bennett's in the labor room. She'll probably deliver in another two or three hours.''

"Already?" Laurie asked. "My God, is there an epidemic of premature labor?''

"She's thirty-eight-and-a-half weeks," Trish said. "That's early, but it's not premature. She's fine. She had both her girls right around thirty-nine weeks. But her husband's out of town. He was coming back tomorrow. She's heartbroken about it, so I came down to hold her hand.''

"You think they'd let me say hello to her?" Laurie asked, hoisting herself up to a sitting position.

Trish's eyes grew wide, and she put her hands out. "Down," she commanded. "Lie back down. Don't you dare try to get up yet. Don't even *think* about getting up.''

Laurie frowned, but she lay back down. "Not even in a wheelchair?" she asked.

"Not even in a wheelchair. I don't want to take any chances. Dr. Crenshaw says you can come to class next week if you stay off your feet for all this next week, *and* if your cervix feels okay that day. But right now, you're on complete bed rest, bedpans and all. I'll tell Norma you said good luck." With a wave of her hand, Trish left. Laurie growled as she switched the television back on.

When it was finally time to leave the hospital the next morning, the nurses allowed Laurie to stand up long enough to put on the clothes she'd been wearing when she arrived, but that was all. No amount of arguing and cajoling could convince them to let her walk a single unnecessary step. Fuming, Laurie let the nurses help her into a wheelchair. They wheeled her out of her room, but instead of taking her down the hallway, they wheeled her into the adjacent room. There, propped up in bed, breastfeeding a bright-red infant, was Norma Bennett. The man Laurie recognized as her husband was standing by the bed. They both looked very tired, and indecently happy.

"Laura Edwards, this is Big Mac," she said, nodding her head toward her husband, "and this," she said, "is Little Mac, who was nine pounds four ounces. Not very little at all." She held the baby out so Laurie could see the tiny face, which instantly contorted into a howl. Norma moved the baby back to her breast, and it contentedly resumed nursing.

"I'm sorry to hear you missed the show," Laurie said to Mac.

"I didn't," he said with a grin.

"He didn't," his wife echoed. "You know what this crazy man did? He chartered a goddam plane! From Cleveland! He got here about twenty minutes before the baby was born. He won't tell me how much it cost."

"Irrelevant," Mac said, still smiling. "Worth twice the price."

"So he misses all the hard part," Norma continued, "and gets here just in time to start yelling 'push!' I coulda hit him."

"You did," Mac said. "Several times."

"Yeah, well you deserved it, whatever it was for."

The nurse standing behind Laurie's wheelchair interrupted. "We'd better go; your husband's waiting downstairs."

Suddenly Norma's face clouded. "I hope you're going to be okay. How do you feel?"

"Fine. They said it was a urinary infection. I have to stay off my feet awhile, but everybody says I shouldn't have any more problems." The nurse began wheeling Laurie out of the room.

"Hang in there," Norma called out as the wheelchair moved out into the hallway.

The ride out of the hospital was long, slow, and ignoble. People would glance at her, then quickly look away. Laurie couldn't remember when she'd felt so awkward, or so embarrassed.

Bill was waiting in the driveway at the main entrance, and he and the nurse gingerly helped Laurie into the front seat of Bill's car, after Laurie flatly refused to get in the back seat and lie down. Enough, she said, was enough.

Once they got home, Bill installed her in the guest room and forbade her to climb the stairs. He'd arranged for their part-time maid to work full-time for the next few weeks, and the maid would do any fetching that needed to be done. Bill was adamant on the subject. Laurie was to stay in bed, period. She could get up to pee, and that was it.

"What about 'number two'?" she asked with sarcastic innocence.

"You know what I mean," he said. "This is no time to be hard-headed. Just stay off your feet."

"Yes, sir," she said dutifully, climbing onto the bed.

Bill put down the armload of belongings he'd been carrying, sat down on the bed beside her, and kissed her. "I don't mean to sound so bossy—well, I guess really I do—but I just feel terrible about this. I feel like it's my fault."

"It *is* your fault," she said with a straight face. "You don't think this is any of *my* doing, do you?'' She let the comment hang in the air a few seconds, enjoying Bill's surprised expression. "Seriously, it's not your fault. It's not mine either, except that I had a bladder infection. But everybody from Dr. Crenshaw down to the busboys has been trying to reassure me that making love had nothing to do with it, except that it helped us notice it then instead of too late.''

"I know,'' Bill said. "I got the same lectures. They're right, of course, but I still feel bad.''

"Good. You should. You're a beast. It's all your fault. You're the one who got me pregnant in the first place, you animal. Gee, I feel better already. This is fun. What's for dinner?''

"Humble pie. Extra portions.''

[19]

Childbirth Classes

IN ALL THE MONTHS of her pregnancy, the only serious argument Laurie had with Bill was over the pillowcases.

Laurie spent one entire week in bed; she ate there, watched television there, read there, slept there. Bill was adamant about not letting her get out of bed. The first day was luxury, of a sort. Laurie reveled in the enforced laziness, watched another episode of one of the soap operas she'd seen in the hospital, and slept. Bill set a kitchen timer on the nightstand, and every four hours, when it rang, Laurie took a Ritodrine tablet and reset the timer.

The second day, the bed started to feel grimy and uncomfortable. The maid obligingly changed the sheets while Laurie took a quick shower and changed nightgowns. That helped for about two hours. Then the bed began to feel lumpy. There was no position that was comfortable, and Laurie shifted back and forth between lying on her left side and her right side. She tried lying on her back, but the pressure of the baby made it uncomfortable. All her life she'd slept on her stomach; that was out of the question now. She read the morning paper from cover to cover, including the classified ads. She tried to watch television but lost interest. She worried at a novel and couldn't concentrate. She tried to conjure up her favorite fantasies and even that didn't work. The boredom was pervasive, all-encompassing, and it was beginning to be painful. She found herself becoming angry at the baby for causing all this mess, then immediately felt guilty for having hostile feelings toward the baby.

In desperation, she called her office and spoke to one of her partners. Yes, he said, there was some work piling up, mostly proposed business deals that she needed to review for any possible antitrust problems, but they could wait; the clients all knew what the delay was about, and could hardly object . . .

Laurie interrupted him. "How many cases are we talking about?" she asked.

The attorney paused, counting. "Seven," he finally announced.

"Put them in a box and send them out here by messenger," she instructed. The man started to protest, but she cut him off. "If I spend one more day in this bed with nothing to do, I'll go nuts and those cases will *never* get read. You don't understand. This won't be work; this is therapy."

The managing partner and a junior associate personally delivered the paperwork, which filled two boxes. They also brought a wheeled library cart to put all the stuff on. Laurie, taken by surprise, told the maid to stall the visitors while she made a forbidden extra trip to the bathroom and arranged her hair, slipped on an embroidered white silk housedress, and arranged the bedcovers neatly before getting back into bed.

The two lawyers were chatty and solicitous and brought her up to date on all the current business and gossip at the firm. The managing partner launched into a long speech assuring Laurie that while they were grateful that she was willing to review all this material now, there was certainly no compelling urgency about any of it, and it could certainly wait, especially if she was going to be back at work in another week or two anyway.

"No guarantees," Laurie said. "But there's no reason I can't do this stuff at home. And I *want* something useful to do. I'm going crazy from the boredom."

The lawyers left, finally, and Laurie discovered that she was exhausted. She rearranged the pillows and napped for an hour. The Ritodrine alarm woke her, and though she tried to go back to sleep after that, the bed had grown uncomfortable again; so, after tossing and turning for a few minutes, she propped herself up on pillows and reached for one of the huge case folders.

Two hours later, when Bill got home, she was utterly absorbed in the case. She was almost annoyed when Bill interrupted her. Then, as her mind withdrew itself from the intricacies of antitrust law, she suddenly realized two things: She wasn't bored any longer, and she desperately needed to pee.

The week passed quickly. Laurie read through all the cases and dictated lengthy memos on each. She kept meticulous track of the time she spent on each; therapy or no therapy, the clients would be billed for her work. When all seven of the cases were complete, she had the maid gather up all the stacks of paper, put them back in the boxes and send them, with her Dictaphone tapes, back to the office. She called the managing partner and told him to send over the next batch.

She consulted her calendar. Tomorrow was the day she was to go back to Crenshaw for her checkup, and, afterward, to her first childbirth class. Damn! They had to take two pillows to the class, and she didn't have any extras in the house.

In defiance of all the orders from Crenshaw and Bill, Laurie got up, showered, and dressed. She walked outside for the first time in a week, got in her car and drove to her favorite department store, where she bought two brand-new pillows and a matched pair of pillowcases.

In retrospect, it was difficult to tell whether Bill had been more upset over her defiance of Crenshaw's (and his) orders to stay in bed, or over the proposition that they should attend childbirth classes equipped with two brand-new pillows in matching designer cases. In the short term, it almost didn't matter. Bill had simply blown up. He used words like "irresponsible" and "arrogant" and "juvenile." When he ran out of intelligent epithets, he started swearing.

To a lawyer, an adversary's anger is a weapon to be turned against him, and Laurie parried thrust after verbal thrust with good humor, until Bill shouted that she was unfit to bear children. Then her own anger flared, instantaneously, beyond hope of control, and she joined the battle with the full fury of all her pent-up frustrations.

It was the kind of fight they later came to reckon time by. The latter part of Laurie's pregnancy was divided into what occurred before the fight and what occurred after. It was, for both of them, the kind of safety-valve experience that is occasionally necessary in an enduring marriage. Just as an earthquake restores equilibrium to the tortured landscape, an all-out conjugal brawl brings balance to a marriage, because it forces into the open all the secret grievances and grudges that accumulate in any relationship.

Laurie and Bill spewed torrents of abuse at each other; they rehashed old iniquities and recited new ones. They blustered and stormed and swore, and occasionally they sniffled. After a full quarter hour, they ran out of fury, and the argument petered out awkwardly. They both felt slightly ashamed of themselves but neither of them was in a position to apologize at that point. Bill simply left the room quietly, leaving Laurie to sulk in bed. After a while, Bill stuck his head in the door. "You gotta eat something," he said quietly.

"I know," Laurie replied, without enthusiasm.

A few minutes later, Bill brought Laurie a tray containing one of his "quick" dinners—braised pork medallions, wild rice, broccoli with hollandaise sauce, a croissant. It was one of Laurie's favorites, and she recognized it as a peace offering. Bill brought a TV tray and they ate together, in silence.

After he cleared the trays away, Bill came back. "I have to go to work real early tomorrow, so I'm going to sleep upstairs tonight. Do you need anything?"

"No."

"Don't forget your pill."

"I won't."

There was a long pause. "I, uh . . . " Bill finally said, awkwardly, "I, uh . . . " His face began to flush slightly.

"I know," Laurie finally interrupted. "Me too. Goodnight."

There was no further mention of pillows or pillowcases. Bill got home in time to drive Laurie to the hospital for her checkup, and he found that Laurie had put the two new pillows on the guest bed and had set two old ones aside, in old but clean pillowcases, for the childbirth class.

Laurie's appointment was at four o'clock, and Bill waited dutifully outside the examining room while Dr. Crenshaw checked Laurie and pronounced her fit to attend the class. She should stay in bed, whenever possible, for another week, he cautioned, but after that she could resume a limited work schedule. "Just be sensible," he cautioned. "No strains, no overexertions. If we can keep you just the way you are for another four or five weeks, we can discontinue the Ritodrine, and you can have your baby any time after that."

There was time to kill between the exam and the class, so Laurie and Bill walked to a nearby restaurant. They were extra polite during dinner; neither of them acknowledged that there had ever been a fight, but the memory of it was fresh enough that it made conversation difficult. Laurie had to sit sideways at the table to keep from bumping against its edge, and after twice dipping a sleeve into her plate, she commented wistfully that although being pregnant was a great experience and she wasn't sorry at all for it, she was going to be awful goddam glad to be done with it.

Bill leaned forward. "What," he asked slowly and conspiritorially, "is the first thing you want to do after you have the baby?"

Laurie paused, staring at her plate as if in deep thought. Then she looked up at Bill with her best poker face. "Deliver the placenta," she said with deadpan earnestness. She watched Bill wince. "Seriously, I don't know," she added. "I think I just want to spend some time getting used to being a mommy."

"Yeah," Bill said with a sigh. "I guess we have to start reading Dr. Spock, or whatever. I know a lot about insurance and not much about raising a kid. What the hell are we going to do?"

"I dunno. I really don't know. I worry about that sometimes."

"Well, let's see. Where should we send him to college?"

"Him? We'll send *her* to Vassar."

"Vassar doesn't have a football team. We'll send *him* to Princeton."

"Pooh. What about names. How does Melissa sound?"

"How about Michael?"

"What makes you so sure it's a boy? Do you know something I don't know?" She glared at him through narrowed eyes.

"Nope. I'm just rooting for my side. How do you like Daniel?"

"Not as much as Donna. Tell you what: If it's a boy, you pick the name, and vice versa. Deal?"

"Deal." Bill looked at his watch. "Time to go. We've got to go learn how to have a baby."

The first childbirth class is always an awkward thing in the beginning, and the class Laurie and Bill attended was no exception. There were four couples, all equipped with pillows, and one couple had also brought a sleeping bag. They met in a medium-size, carpeted room in the private office suite at the hospital. All four of the women seemed hugely pregnant, and all four of the men appeared profoundly uncomfortable.

Trish looked around the room. Some classes were easier than others, and small classes were usually the easiest. It was simply a matter of getting the ice broken. "I think I know everybody here, but just in case, my name is Trish," she began. "Let's go around the room and get everybody else's name, starting over here." She pointed at Laurie and Bill, who obligingly announced their names. The other three couples followed suit. Laurie watched each of the faces in turn. The couple sitting next to them, Linda and Woodie Meyer, seemed to be closest to Laurie's age; early-to-mid thirties, Laurie guessed. Next to them sat a much younger couple named Alice and Dwight King. The couple at the far right of the semicircle gave their names as Jill Hardaway and Robert Harrison, and instantly the eyes of the other three couples dropped to inspect their hands for wedding rings. They had them. The uncomfortable silence returned.

Trish continued. "I'm here to try to give you the knowledge and the preparation you need to make your birth experience a really positive one. Now I want to go around the room again, and I want to ask each one of you why you're here, and I want to know the real reasons. Guys, if you're here because she dragged you here, then say that. If you women are only here because your doctors told you to, then let's hear that. We're going to be really frank and really blunt in these classes, and this is a good time to start. Now,'' she said pointing, ''why are you here?''

''She dragged me,'' Woodie Meyer said with a wry grin.

His wife glared at him, then announced, ''We're here because we want a positive birth experience.''

''I agree with that,'' said Alice King. ''Anything that will make it more positive is worth spending time on.''

''We're here because the doctor recommended it, but we're here for us, not him,'' her husband added.

''I want to learn the breathing techniques,'' Jill Hardaway said. ''They say the breathing really helps.''

Robert Harrison shrugged slightly. ''Where she goes, I go,'' he said.

Trish looked back to the other side of the circle, and pointed to Laurie.

''I want to know what to expect,'' she said simply.

''I'm here to learn sensitivity,'' Bill said with a trace of a lisp and a look of angelic innocence. Laurie gritted her teeth, but Trish grinned.

''You mean she dragged you,'' she said, then paused, waiting for a chuckle. One or two people smiled, then the awkward silence settled over the group again.

Trish took a deep breath. Some classes were definitely tougher than others. ''Okay, gang, this next part is going to be easy. We're going to see a movie.''

When a class is especially reticent, Trish knew, the shock treatment was often the best solution. She spent a few minutes fiddling with the projector, then dimmed the lights and sat back to watch, for the umpteenth time, a forty-five-minute film called ''Nan's Class.''

The movie was about, naturally enough, childbirth classes, and it might have been calibrated on a slide rule to provide the maximum number of role models. There was a black couple, a white couple, a Hispanic couple. There was a rich couple and a poor couple, a homely couple and a beautiful couple. There was a single mother, whose partner, or "coach," was a female friend. Something for everyone.

One by one, the couples—and the single mother—all had their babies, in full view of the camera. The "Mr. and Mrs. America" couple surprised everyone when Mrs. America ultimately was delivered by cesarean section. The movie was sprinkled liberally with episiotomies, stitches, placentas, blood, and body fluids. Some of the women suffered more pain than the others, but all of them obviously experienced pain. By the end of the movie, there was nothing about the childbirth experience that had not been shown at least once. In the final scene all the parents gathered in front of the camera to show off their normal, healthy, happy babies.

Trish shut off the projector and turned up the room lights. "Well?" she demanded. "What impressed you most?" She pointed a finger.

"I didn't know babies looked so slimy when they came out," said Jill Hardaway. "What was that stuff all over them?"

"It's a natural protective coating," Trish said. "It's called vernix. If you kept your hand in water for nine months, it'd get pretty shriveled unless you had something on there to protect it. That's what vernix is. It washes right off."

"Why did they do that cesarean section?" asked Linda Meyer.

"They were worried about the baby, and they wanted to get it out right then."

"But why couldn't they just wait? Why not let that woman have a natural childbirth?"

"Okay," Trish said. "Let's think about the reasons they might have for wanting to do a section. Who can think of one?"

"The baby was too big," Dwight King offered.

"Right. That's one. What else?"

"The baby was a breech."

"Good. Everybody knows what breech is? Feet first. You can

deliver a breech baby vaginally, but most doctors like to do C-sections, because it's safer. There's another position called a 'transverse lie' that's worse than breech, where the baby has its back to the birth canal and can't possibly come out. They always do a section for that, and for things like a shoulder presentation. So breech, or other bad position, is another reason to do a section. What else?''

Laurie spoke up. "You said that they were worried about the baby. Why were they worried?"

"Fetal distress," Trish answered, "and that's the next reason. The baby's in trouble. It's not getting enough oxygen for some reason, which means you need to do something quick, before there's any damage. That's what they use the fetal heart monitor for. They can tell how the baby's doing by watching the fetal heartbeat."

"All the babies looked blue when they came out," Alice King said. "Doesn't that mean they weren't getting enough oxygen?"

"Yes, it does," Trish said, "but that's not the same thing as fetal distress. When babies that have been in real distress are born, they're very loose and floppy, they don't cry, and they don't move their arms and legs very much. There's a standard scale, called the Apgar score, which ranks babies from one to ten on how good they look when they're born. Zero is no vital signs, and it's very bad. Ten is perfect; only the children of pediatricians have Apgar scores of ten." She paused, and there were a few chuckles, at last.

"But to get back to your question, a lot of babies are not all pink when they're born; the hands and feet of most of them are blue for the first couple of minutes. That's because their whole circulatory system is changing right then, from using the mother's oxygen supply to using their own. It usually takes a couple of minutes for them to get used to it, and that's why they're a little bit blue. But that's not the same as fetal distress. They turn pink after a few minutes."

"They all looked deformed," Alice King continued. "Did you see their heads? They all looked like little coneheads."

"They do that for your benefit," Trish answered. "The reason you go into labor when you do is because the baby has gotten as big as he can get and still make it through the birth canal. And the toughest thing to get through that canal is the baby's head. The reason the baby's head is shaped that way is because the plates that make up his skull aren't all fused together yet, which makes the skull more flexible, and it actually elongates to make it pass through the birth canal more easily. It goes back to a more rounded shape within a day or two."

The questions continued a few minutes longer, until finally Trish called a halt. "We've only got about fifteen minutes left," she said, "and there's one more thing we need to get started on, because it's something you need to practice at home, too. Have any of you done relaxation techniques before?"

There were blank stares. "Believe it or not, relaxation is one of the most important things you'll be doing when you're in labor," Trish went on, "and it's something we want to start practicing right from the first. That's one of the things you brought the pillows for."

Relaxation, it turned out, was done lying down. There was some general shuffling around as the couples arranged themselves on the floor. The women stretched out supine, their heads and shoulders elevated by the pillows, to make breathing a little easier. The men crouched, knelt, or sat cross-legged beside them.

"What we're going to do now is to practice consciously relaxing everything, every part of the body," Trish said, her voice lapsing into a soothing, singsong rhythm. She stretched the word *relax*, savored it each time she spoke it, let the final syllable hang in the air an extra millisecond every time she said it.

"We'll start by relaxing just one side of your body, relaxing just one arm and one leg. Tighten them up, make a fist, tighten your muscles, really tight, and then let them both go limp, let them relax.

"Now," she directed the men. "Take her elbow with one hand and her wrist with the other and lift her arm. Feel how heavy it is? If it's not heavy, she's not relaxed. Now try it again, on the other side this time."

The exercises continued, with Trish encouraging the women to relax and coaching the husbands on how to help. "Look at her face," she said. "If she's smiling, she's not relaxed. Relax. Relaaaaaaaaax."

About five minutes before quitting time, Trish pulled her favorite switch. "Okay," she said, "now that the women have all had a chance to try this, let's turn the tables. I want the men to lie down and try the same relaxation techniques."

It took several minutes to rearrange positions, and then the men lay on the pillows, their wives beside them. All four men relaxed quickly and completely. Their bodies became heavy and flaccid, their faces went slack and their breathing slowed to four times a minute.

"That's very good," Trish complimented them. "Both of you should practice that at home this next week. And the men should be better at it than the women. You know why?" she asked. There was a chorus of nos.

"Two main reasons," she continued. "The first is that you guys don't have an extra twenty pounds sitting on your stomach, so it's easier to do the deep breathing. The other is that you know you're not the one that's going to be in labor. So it's a lot easier for you to relax.

"Do the relaxation this week," she repeated, "and next week we'll start working on breathing techniques."

"Well, was that so bad?" Laurie demanded of Bill as they walked to the parking garage.

"Golly no," Bill said in his sincerest voice. "I feel so sensitive now." He dodged as Laurie tried to jab him in the ribs. "Seriously, it wasn't bad. I do feel a little guilty, though, when I realize that you've got all the tough parts of this business. I don't know why you think having me there will help any, but if you want it, you've got it."

"Oh, I just want you to feel guilty for the rest of your life," Laurie said airily. "Besides, this is going to be a real show. You wouldn't want to miss it."

[20]

The Gong Test

LAURIE stayed in bed most of the following week, and once or twice she and Bill dutifully practiced the relaxation techniques Trish had taught them. Crenshaw had told Laurie to phone if she noticed any changes and had scheduled another exam for the afternoon that she'd have childbirth class.

Her partners in the law firm seemed pleased with her part-time working arrangement, and certainly Laurie was grateful for the distraction. She'd led an active life for thirty-nine years now, and being confined in bed was as bad as being confined in jail. Worse, she decided. There was no appeal from the bed-rest order.

There was no longer a strict prohibition against getting up, but Laurie tried hard to stay off her feet. Once or twice she moved to a chaise lounge in the back yard and basked in the sunshine, but for the most part she stayed indoors. The maid had gone back to a part-time schedule, and Laurie was secretly grateful; now she felt less like an invalid. She still inhabited the guest bedroom to avoid climbing the stairs, although she had made the forbidden trip once, to retrieve a law book she particularly needed and to prove to herself she could do it. The effort left her winded, but there were no contractions.

She still took the Ritodrine religiously every four hours. Crenshaw said it was a precaution; the contractions probably wouldn't start again, since her last urine specimen had been infection-free, but why take a chance? If she went into premature labor again, the chances of stopping it would be less than before, and she had come far too close to having the baby the first time. Laurie was now thirty-three weeks pregnant, almost thirty-four. If she delivered the baby that day, the baby would almost surely survive, but there would be a long, agonizing month while the child lived in the artificial womb of the intensive-care nursery. Every extra day that the baby stayed inside Laurie was one less day in the preemie ward. So, without fail, every four hours, day and night, the alarm sounded and Laurie took a pill.

Every time he saw her, Crenshaw warned her to watch for all the possible side effects of the Ritodrine—the sudden nervousness, the ringing in the ears, the dizziness—and to report them instantly if she felt them. Improving the baby's odds was fine, he said, but only if it didn't damage Laurie.

Bill left for work early and came home early on the day they were to attend childbirth class. He again sat in the waiting room while Crenshaw checked Laurie and pronounced everything fine. They had another leisurely dinner in a downtown restaurant, and conducted a spirited debate over what a boy-child would accomplish as opposed to a girl-child. The issue remained unresolved.

In the class, Trish introduced them to breathing techniques. They could as easily be called yoga techniques, she said, or meditation techniques, or even autohypnosis. There were nearly as many breathing techniques as there were childbirth class instructors, she explained, and most of them seemed to work equally well.

"It really breaks down into two parts," she explained. "During early labor, the first stage, you do the slow, deep breathing, because you're trying to relax. The more you can relax, the more your cervix can relax, and the more your cervix can relax, the more rapidly labor can proceed. Then in the second stage, when you're actually having the baby, you take shallow, panting breaths during the contractions, so you're not adding any extra pressure from your diaphragm.

"But I always tell people to do whatever kind of breathing they're most comfortable with, because that's what it's for, to make labor less uncomfortable. It'll still hurt, but it won't be unbearable. People who've done it both ways say the relaxation makes the pain a lot easier to tolerate.

"Don't think there's not going to be some pain, though. There will be. This is simply one way to deal with it."

"Why doesn't everybody have a spinal block?" asked Robert Harrison.

Trish made a face. "Oh, anesthesia! Why does everybody need an epidural? What's wrong with pain? We're all brainwashed as children, taught that the minute you have pain it's a bad thing. I've watched a lot of women deliver, and there's nothing more exciting than someone delivering without having had any anesthesia. It's such a high, and it's so vivid, and so clear."

She paused for a moment. "That is not to say that anesthesia is inappropriate in every case," she added. "If a woman's been in labor for thirty hours and she's exhausted, an epidural can be just what she needs for that last big push. But it's an individual thing. It's really not for everyone."

The back-and-forth continued for more than an hour. It was almost as though it was a different group; the reserve of the previous week was gone. The questions came in a steady flow, and covered a great number of delicate and indelicate matters.

At the University of Maryland Hospital, Trish explained, laboring mothers were no longer shaved. Many hospitals continued the practice, but study after study had showed that it made no difference in the infection rate for either the mother or the baby, so Dr. Crenshaw had decreed that the practice stop. A woman in labor had enough annoyances already, without that indignity.

The same was true for enemas, she said. The guiding philosophy behind enemas had been the same as shaving: to prevent infection. Once again, studies had showed it made no difference, so another undignified annoyance had been dispensed with. And yet, she added, that too was still a requirement at many hospitals. "I've talked to women who honestly thought you couldn't have a baby without having an enema first," she said. Besides, she added, early in labor the pressure on the large intestine intensifies, and the bowels tend to move of their own accord. "Don't worry about it one way or the other," Trish counseled. "That's something that takes care of itself."

Something that did not take care of itself, and something that concerned many of the women that night, was episiotomies and stitches. Trish answered the question cautiously. "There's a lot of controversy about episiotomies. A lot of the more radical types say that doctors cut episiotomies just for their own convenience, even when they don't really have to. I don't know if that's true or not other places; I can only speak for this hospital, where it's not.

"But it is definitely a judgment call on the doctor's part. If the doctor thinks you're about to tear, then he's going to want to cut an episiotomy. Now, that is, in one sense, for his convenience, because then he only has one place to sew up. If you tear naturally, you'll probably tear in several places, and he's got to sew them up, one at a time.

"And that's why I always say that an episiotomy is for *your* convenience more than the doctor's. Stitches are not fun." She paused a moment. "No, let me rephrase that. Stitches hurt like hell. I've had women say the labor wasn't bad, and even the delivery wasn't too bad, but the stitches were horrible. But if, for whatever reason, you absolutely without question don't want an episiotomy, then tell the doctor that, both of you, and he'll honor the request."

The discussion went on, then, into the nature, type, and philosophy of episiotomies. The purpose of an episiotomy, Trish explained, is to widen the introitus at that last critical moment when the baby's head is forcing its way out. By making a small cut either directly at the bottom or on either or both sides of the introitus, the physician is able to add that extra capacity to the birth canal before it tears of its own accord at the weakest place. The episiotomy controls the direction and usually also the extent of the wound; without the episiotomy, the tearing often extends to some of the more significant muscles in the perineum, the region where the thighs meet, and healing is then slower and more painful.

From episiotomies the conversation progressed to cesarean sections, and when and how often they should be done. Trish tackled the subject head-on.

"A section is sort of the ultimate precaution," she said. "It's fast, it's reliable and, as surgery goes, it's safe. If an obstetrician has any doubt at all about how that baby's doing, he's going to be thinking about the possibility of a section. Some doctors probably carry that to extremes. But obstetricians are never sued for doing sections; the're sued for *not* doing them when they should have.

"So here's the obstetrician caught in the middle. He's sued for not doing sections, so he does more sections, and then he's criticized for doing too many sections. Once again, I can't speak for any place but UMH, but I can tell you that here they try to avoid doing sections whenever possible.

"Sometimes it's obvious that you have to do a section: The baby is a shoulder presentation, and you have no choice. Sometimes you may think the baby's too big, and then the mother delivers just fine. So you can't always be sure. You try to be cautious.

"The fuzziest area is fetal distress. If we start seeing late decelerations on the fetal-heart monitor, that may mean the baby's in distress and it may not. Now, that's where you get most of your sections that people later say may not have been necessary. That's always easier to say after the fact, of course, and some of them probably were unnecessary. But when an obstetrician sees the late decelerations, and he knows that in a certain percentage of all cases those late decelerations mean the baby's in serious trouble, what's he going to do? What would you want him to do?

"Now that brings up one of the advantages of having a baby in a tertiary-care center like this one. Because this is a large teaching hospital, we have more resources instantly available to us than you would find at the ordinary community hospital. If a doctor at the community hospital starts seeing late decelerations, and he knows that from the time he decides to do a section it's going to take half an hour to get the OR set up, he has to make his decision right away.

"Here, if we have to do a section, we can be ready in five minutes, and that gives us more time to think about it. We can make the decision more carefully, and gather more information before we make the decision, without endangering the baby. So at this hospital, if we start seeing late decelerations and we're worried that the baby may be in trouble, we do something called a fetal scalp pH, where we take a blood sample from the baby's scalp and test to see if it's too acid. If it is, that means the baby really is having trouble. If the blood is okay, then we know the baby's okay. If it's not, then it's time for a section.

"And that's something you all have to be prepared for," she said, looking around the room. "There's no way to predict ahead of time who's going to need a section. Most people don't need one, but, just like in the movie last week, suddenly there it is and you have to make a decision quickly.

"You have to try to be as open-minded about it as possible, and not just about the section—about medications, the monitor, epidurals, and the whole high-tech experience. Ideally, you want to avoid all those things, but realistically, you know you're not going to let your baby die. You know that. You'll do anything for your baby, and that includes medicines, monitoring, even a C-section."

The discussion continued awhile longer, then Trish reined it in. "We were originally talking about breathing techniques, and we ought to practice them now."

It was difficult not to be self-conscious during the breathing exercises. The men squatted or sat cross-legged beside their wives while the women practiced the deep-breathing techniques they would use early in labor, then the shorter and quicker ones for the later stages. Since the average contraction lasts about sixty seconds, the breathing exercises were timed to last one minute.

Laurie considered the exercises tedious and a little elementary; she'd been involved in athletic activities of one sort or another since high school, and she knew how to make her lungs work at maximum efficiency. That was really the point to all this, she thought. But she kept quiet and breathed dutifully on command. She was relieved when the session finally ended.

The visits to the hospital settled into a weekly routine, for checkup and classes. The following week, Crenshaw told Laurie she could resume working half-days. In class, they talked about the placenta and practiced breathing. Laurie listened with half an ear.

Much of the work she did at the firm consisted of reviewing business proposals, and that could be done anywhere. But a certain number of face-to-face encounters were necessary, and now that Laurie was able to spend mornings at the firm, she scheduled meetings every half hour from nine to noon. She had her rocking chair moved to the conference room; for some reason, the baby tended to kick more often and more violently if she sat in one of the conference room's high-backed swivel chairs, and that often made it difficult to carry on a conversation. So Laurie rocked while she talked, and it gave the meetings a warmth and informality that was uncharacteristic of the gray pin-striped world of business law, but it seemed to delight Laurie's clients. Indeed, the firm had attracted a great many new clients during Laurie's pregnancy; so many, in fact, that the managing partner had once joked that the firm should offer Laurie a bonus if she would stay pregnant.

Laurie always took case files home with her in the afternoons and, without the distractions of the office, was able to accomplish a great deal of work. She had resumed sleeping upstairs at night, but maintained the guest bedroom as her workplace. There was no place to lie down in her study upstairs.

She had become accustomed to the baby's habits now—even attached to them, after a fashion. The baby, Trish had explained, had its own sleep-wake cycle, and each part usually lasted about an hour. That matched Laurie's own experience. In the beginning, when she'd first been able to feel the baby moving, the movements hadn't seemed to follow any definite pattern, but now she could recognize the pattern right away. She could control it, too. The baby seemed to enjoy motion of any sort; whenever Laurie walked, or rocked in her rocking chair, the baby stayed quiet. If she sat still in a chair, or lay quiet in bed, the baby seemed to get restless. First there would be a couple of light touches, as though the baby was stretching, and then would come a series of intermittent blows, some hard enough to take her breath away. It was as though the baby was pounding its fist, saying "C'mon, rock me some more." The idea fascinated

Laurie, and she tried walking around when the baby got restless. It seemed to work, but it was of limited value; Laurie always tired out before the baby did.

Dr. Crenshaw was out of town the following week. While Dr. Nagey examined Laurie, she explained her conclusions about the baby's movement. Nagey nodded his head. "That's probably exactly what's going on," he agreed. "The kid was pounding on my stethoscope a minute ago. You know the most fascinating thing to me about that sleep-wake cycle is that apparently they dream."

"They what?"

"They dream—or at least they do the same things you and I do when we dream. They have REM sleep. You know, the rapid eye movements? People do that when they're dreaming. Somebody did a big ultrasound study and showed that unborn babies have REM cycles when they sleep."

"Jeez," Laurie said appreciatively. "That's amazing."

"Isn't it? Who knows what they dream about." He paused, then added, "Your cervix feels terrific, by the way. If I hadn't read your chart, I'd have a hard time guessing that you almost had this baby five weeks ago."

Laurie and Bill had dinner at yet another restaurant that evening; it had been a long time since they'd explored restaurants together. For Laurie it was the highlight of the evening; she was beginning to get restless in the childbirth classes. She had been reading about childbirth for seven months and while the movie had rounded out her academic knowledge, she now found much of the discussion elementary. Oddly, Bill seemed to be enjoying himself, as did the other three men. The men asked most of the questions that night, and the questions were mostly about their role as coach in the childbirth process.

"I will take your word for it that what we'll be doing is important," Woodie Meyer said, "and certainly I'm not going to pass up the chance to be there, but frankly, I must be the least qualified person you could find for the job."

"You're probably right," Trish grinned at him, drawing a chuckle from the rest of the class. "Except," she added, "for one or two little things. She," Trish pointed to Woodie's wife Linda, "loves you. She trusts you. She knows you and knows you love her. The rest of the people in the delivery room are going to be strangers, more or less, so just having you there for the company makes it worthwhile.

"But you do more than that. Right at the last, when the baby's ready to come out, things are happening fast, and Linda won't have much time to think. If you say 'push,' she will respond quicker and push harder than she will for a stranger, because she knows without thinking about it that you're on her side.

"That's the real reason you're there. Strictly speaking, it doesn't have to be you; it could be anybody she knows and loves and trusts. Some single mothers bring their own mothers or their sisters. But women who have coaches have, on the average, shorter labors and easier deliveries than women who don't. It's a purely psychological thing. Childbirth is an intensely personal experience, and it goes better if you know you're among friends."

The conversation turned to episiotomies, and Laurie's attention began to drift. Her one bright spot in the two-hour class came later, when she discussed her discovery of the sleep-wake cycle and the possibility that unborn babies dream. Trish nodded approvingly, and Laurie's classmates expressed varying degrees of excitement and wonder.

That night, Laurie got the first uninterrupted night's sleep she'd had in five weeks. Nagey had told her she could stop taking the Ritodrine. Her cervix had firmed up remarkably well and her infection was gone, apparently for good. But most important of all, it didn't matter anymore. She was thirty-six weeks pregnant now, and if she went into labor, she would have a baby. From here it was all downhill.

Laurie began making all the standard preparations, heeding some of the advice she'd gotten from her mother, Bill's mother, and, it sometimes seemed, every other woman she'd ever known.

She packed a small duffel bag with a few essentials, including three back issues of law-review journals she hadn't gotten around to reading. She packed a bathrobe, but no nightgown. From her previous stay there, she knew the hospital preferred that patients wear the perverse little open-backed gowns. She packed her own soap, her own shampoo and toothpaste. She bought an extra toothbrush and stowed it in the bag.

She made sure there was plenty of film for their camera and mailers for the film. She wrote the addresses on the mailers and put stamps on them. She began filling her gas tank whenever it dropped to half full. After talking to two friends who'd had children, she switched to a larger purse so she could discreetly carry several superabsorbent sanitary napkins, in case her water broke without warning.

She went to work every morning; she conducted rocking-chair meetings, though less frequently than at first. In the afternoons, she read voraciously, usually in bed, during what she had come to think of as her "quiet time." The baby participated in Laurie's quiet time by performing drum rolls, complete with ruffles and flourishes, on her diaphragm.

One afternoon, Laurie dozed off as she read a particularly boring corporate reorganization plan and slept for a little over an hour. She awoke needing desperately to urinate, which seemed like her normal state with the baby so large and pressing against her bladder all the time. When she got back in bed, she resumed reading. She was a little bemused that she had actually fallen asleep. Not that she wasn't tired; she felt tired all the time lately, but the baby usually kept her awake.

That *was* odd, now that she thought about it. The baby had been very quiet that afternoon. Very quiet indeed, considering she hadn't been moving around much at all. She waited, paying close attention. Sure enough, the baby wasn't moving.

Well, she thought, if she was tired, so was the baby, no doubt. She got back out of bed, walked to the kitchen, and poured a glass of milk. She slowly paced the length of the kitchen as she drank the milk, then went back to the guest bedroom and lay quiet again, waiting for the baby to move. She glanced at the clock radio. It was a few minutes after three. She picked up the document she'd been reading, tried to read more of it, but kept glancing at the clock. When the baby still hadn't moved by three-thirty, she reached for the phone.

The answering service took her phone number, and within minutes Dr. Pupkin phoned. "This is probably very silly," Laurie said, "but the baby hasn't been moving as much as usual. I haven't felt anything at all for the last forty-five minutes or so, and I slept for about an hour before that, which means there couldn't have been much movement. I usually wake up if there is. Am I being paranoid?"

"Probably," Pupkin answered. "But that's your job. And my job is to be just as cautious. Can you come down here right now? I'll be glad to check you."

Laurie arrived at the hospital just before the four-o'clock exodus began and had to hunt for a parking place. She'd felt a couple of movements, and that reassured her that she was indeed being overcautious; but still, the baby wasn't being as vigorous as usual, and that was certainly cause for alarm. Or if not alarm, at least it was cause to make sure everything was functioning properly.

In the field of obstetrics, nothing rivals the placenta for sheer lack of glamour. Placentas, the medical students learn from the residents, are boring. And ugly. And messy. When, in the golden moments following delivery, everyone clusters around the mother to admire the newborn, it is the most junior member of the delivery-room team who stands alone at the foot of the bed, a gloved hand idly clutching the freshly-cut umbilical cord as though it were a leash leading back through the birth canal to some stubborn creature not yet willing to come out of the womb. Nobody takes much interest in placentas.

But the placenta is unique in all of mammalian physiology. It is the world's only disposable organ: a single-use, no-deposit, no-return biological engine. And it is remarkably complex.

In a sense it is a parasite, since it siphons off oxygen and nutrients from the mother's blood supply and dumps metabolic waste products in their place. In another sense it is a symbiont, since it produces hormones that interact with the mother's hormones to maintain a stable pregnancy. But most important of all, the placenta, together with the fetal membranes, provides a miniature incubator, a protected environment in which new life can form.

In the true fashion of a disposable organ, the placenta is not designed for durability. A heart, or a kidney, is built to last a lifetime; on the average, a placenta need last only forty weeks.

Nature's design specifications for the placenta cut close to that line. By forty weeks, most placentas begin to show signs of deterioration. At forty-two weeks, obstetricians start to become alarmed; like an out-of-warranty automobile, a forty-two-week placenta is not to be trusted. Most obstetricians will induce labor at forty-two weeks rather than trust the placenta to last forty-three.

There is only one test that, theoretically, can tell with certainty whether a placenta is working properly, a test that Dr. Pupkin and Dr. Nagey invented when they were still at Duke. It is time-consuming, cumbersome, and expensive. The mother is given an injection of a chemical that the placenta usually metabolizes rapidly. Then her blood is checked periodically to see how quickly the chemical dissipates. If it dissipates in a short time, the placenta is working fine; if not, there is a problem.

When Pupkin and Nagey reported the test in the professional literature, it generated a great deal of excitement in the scientific community, but it did not arouse much interest among practitioners. For all its scientific merit, the test was not practical. It took too long and cost too much. Besides, there were other tests available that, while not true placental-function tests, served much the same purpose.

The simplest of the tests involved placing a fetal-heart monitor on the mother's abdomen and giving her a button to push whenever the baby moved. The theory behind the test was elegantly simple: When the baby moved, its heart rate should speed up. Exercise should affect the fetus the same way it affects an adult.

If, however, the placenta wasn't functioning properly, and the baby was sluggish from lack of oxygen, the heart rate might go up less, or not at all. Fetal movement that was not accompanied by an increased heart rate was cause for concern. But it was not cause for alarm. The test often gave false positives—what Dr. Nagey liked to call the "absence of reassurance." If the results of the test were not reassuring, there was another test, more reliable but also more risky.

Just as fetal movement will accelerate the heartbeat, a uterine contraction can slow it down if the baby is not getting enough oxygen. During a contraction, the arteries that supply fresh blood to the placenta are squeezed shut. If the placenta is functioning properly, there is a supply of oxygen-laden blood already inside the organ, more than enough to sustain the baby for the minute or so that the contraction lasts.

When a placenta has begun to deteriorate, that margin is reduced, and a contraction can cause a significant reduction in the baby's oxygen supply. When that happens, the baby's heartbeat will slow either during the contraction or right after it, will remain slow for several seconds, and will then return slowly back to normal, as the oxygen level rises in the fetal bloodstream.

It is not the "late deceleration" itself that causes an obstetrician to become anxious; it is the slowness with which the baby's heartbeat returns to normal. It is that long, flat curve that, in theory, demonstrates that the baby is in distress.

In practice, it is not so simple, and the validity of the fetal heart monitor in predicting fetal distress is one of the hottest continuing debates in all of obstetrics. Many obstetricians will perform emergency cesarean sections at the first sign of late decelerations. Many of the babies thus delivered show no obvious signs of having been in distress, though, and there is one school of thought which says the C-section was not necessary. The other school of thought says the baby got out just in the nick of time, before anything went seriously wrong.

Pupkin and his colleagues at the University of Maryland have heard both sides of the argument, and they know that the answer lies somewhere between the two extremes. The fetal heart monitor, is an imperfect device, but they also know that, on the average, it is a great help.

It was of little use to Laurie at the moment because she was not having contractions. If Pupkin wanted to measure the baby's response to a uterine contraction, it would be necessary to give Laurie a drug called oxytocin, which causes contractions. Pupkin wanted to avoid that if he could; the drug probably wouldn't cause Laurie to go into labor again, but he did not want to take the chance.

The third alternative, thanks to the work of a former chief resident, was what the literature called the "Acoustic Stimulation Nonstress Test," and what everyone at University Hospital called simply the "Gong Test."

The resident, Paolo Serafini, had read about the gong test while he was still a medical student in Rio de Janeiro. When he came to Baltimore to train in obstetrics, he brought with him a small audio amplifier and a black metal cylinder containing a small loudspeaker. The test was simple. Laurie's concern was that the baby wasn't moving. Testing the baby's heart rate required the baby to move. The gong test solved that paradoxical problem by startling the baby with a strange sound.

Pupkin led Laurie to an empty labor room, where a nurse helped her onto one of the beds, then instructed her to rearrange her clothing to expose her abdomen. The nurse then strapped and taped her abdomen with several fetal-heart monitor sensors. The nurse flipped a switch on the machine and it hummed to life, tracing the wavy pattern of the baby's heartbeat on a moving strip of paper.

Pupkin took the "gong" by its handle, held it to his ear, and pressed the button once to make sure it was working. Then he pressed it against Laurie's abdomen, a short distance from the baby's head. By the thirtieth week of pregnancy, a baby's hearing mechanism is fully developed, but all the baby usually hears is the lub-dub, lub-dub, lub-dub of the mother's heart, the gurgling and rumbling of her intestines, and the rhythm of her voice when she speaks. When Pupkin pressed the button on the loudspeaker, a high-pitched whistling noise filled the uterus. It wasn't loud, just unusual and startling.

The baby kicked.

Laurie, taken by surprise, gasped for breath. The baby had scored a direct hit on her diaphragm. Pupkin pressed the button again.

The baby moved again.

"I knew I was being paranoid," Laurie said, breathing shallowly.

Pupkin stood upright, replaced the loudspeaker on top of the amplifier, then tore off the strip of paper that protruded from the fetal heart monitor. He grinned.

"Look here," he said to Laurie, pointing. "Perfect. Every one of them." Each time the baby had moved, the heartbeat had jumped, then settled back. "Your baby's fine."

[21]

It's Time!

THERE IS no scientific definition of the moment when labor begins, but all the textbooks say that active labor is clinically unmistakable and that the first stage consists of "the progressive effacement and dilation of the cervix in response to painful uterine contractions."

If Laurie had learned one thing in childbirth classes, it was to believe that labor would be a painful experience. Trish had not dwelt unnecessarily on the subject, but it came up several times, in several contexts, during each class. Yes, it will be painful, Trish would say, and all the breathing and relaxation in the world won't make it not hurt. What we hope is that you'll see the pain as a natural part of the process and be comfortable with it. Tensing up only makes it worse.

More than once, Trish had used the analogy of ski slopes. "You're at the top of the mountain now, and one way or the other, you're going to get to the bottom. How you do it is really up to you, but the more you're prepared, the easier it will be." Laurie dutifully practiced relaxing during her quiet time in the afternoons, and occasionally she worked, albiet unenthusiastically, on breathing exercises. Somehow, she had difficulty believing that any sort of controlled breathing was going to reduce pain.

Indeed, she still entertained some doubts about just how painful labor would be. She'd been in labor once already, for a while, and the sensations had been, well, unusual—but she would not have described them as painful. To Laurie, pain was the sharp, bright pain of a burnt finger, or the slow relentless agony of a broken arm. Her contractions had been uncomfortable, certainly. To say they were painful was overstating it. She had felt cramped. The last few contractions gave a cramping sort of feeling, the way you feel when you're straining to run one more lap, to do the last four or five sit-ups. It was the sort of sensation you feel the next day when you try to use those sore muscles. She had not felt severely cramped: on a scale of one to ten, a two, perhaps a three at the most.

Laurie was enough of an athlete to be familiar with that sort of pain, and was unafraid of it and more than a little skeptical about the effect of breathing exercises on it. Nevertheless, she dutifully attended the remaining childbirth classes, went through the motions, smiled and nodded at the appropriate times. The last class was held during Laurie's thirty-eighth week; Trish brought refreshments, and an alumnus of an earlier class brought her baby to show off.

Laurie continued to go to work every day, although some mornings it took all her willpower to get out of bed. She was always tired; between the baby and her bladder, she never slept more than an hour at a time. More and more often, she fell asleep during her afternoon quiet time, and she went to bed earlier and earlier at night. She and Bill resumed sleeping in the guest bedroom, not because there was any particular danger in climbing the stairs now, but simply because it was too much work. Sometimes, if they wanted to go upstairs to inspect the baby's room, Bill would get behind Laurie and push.

On Saturday of Laurie's thirty-ninth week, a chilly April day, she and Bill went shopping for baby paraphernalia. Laurie had been adamant about not having a baby shower, so her friends had mailed gifts to her instead. She had received two pairs of flannel baby pajamas, three tiny T-shirts, one flannel blanket, and three toys that made noise. In a two-hour shopping spree, she added four pairs of terrycloth sleepers, three blankets, five pairs of booties, two cartons of disposable diapers, a collection of baby oil and powder and shampoo, cotton balls, cotton swabs, and premoistened towelettes, and six cans and bottles of disinfectants and air fresheners.

Back at the house, they put everything neatly in the baby's room. The shopping episode had been invigorating for Laurie; it was tangible evidence that she was almost "done." Her attitude had begun to shift subtly, so that the pregnancy and the baby were almost separate from each other. The baby existed, in her mind, as a separate person, a person who could come home with her as soon as this job of pregnancy was finished. She craved to touch the baby, to cradle her in her arms and hold her to her breast, and the desire had intensified in the past few weeks. The delivery-room fantasies persisted, but they no longer dwelt on the process; everything centered around the moment when she could caress her baby.

Laurie tried to nap that afternoon, but the baby was restless and so was she. Bill had retreated to his basement shop, where he was assembling shelves to hang on the wall of the baby's room. Laurie had the upstairs to herself. She walked around aimlessly for a while, stopped in the kitchen for a glass of milk, and suddenly decided to cook dinner.

Laurie's cooking tended to be practical, whereas Bill's was elaborate, and she was usually content to leave mealtime to him; but tonight, somehow, she felt like cooking. She found steaks in the freezer, selected two, and started them thawing in the microwave oven. She washed potatoes and put them in the toaster-oven to bake. She rummaged in the refrigerator, took out a variety of salad ingredients from odd places, and assembled a tossed salad, which she put back in the refrigerator.

That done, she found she still had half an hour to wait before the potatoes would be ready. She spent the time rummaging through the pantry, arranging things into a more logical order. Bill came up from the basement just as Laurie was starting to broil the steaks. He protested at Laurie's preparation of dinner and gave all the appropriate compliments to the meal. He looked like he wanted to cry when Laurie proudly showed him how she'd rearranged his pantry, but all he said was, "Aren't you sweet?"

For Laurie's part, she felt robust and full of ginger, ready to fight tigers. She decided she wanted wine—a good, dark hearty red wine. Bill located a bottle of Bordeaux that wasn't quite mature, and Laurie drank two glasses of the raw, flinty wine with the dinner, which Bill had to admit was excellent. After dinner, Laurie decided she wanted ice cream for dessert and then decided she wanted to walk the two blocks to the ice-cream store. Bill was mystified; they hadn't gone for a walk since just before Laurie's premature labor. But he fetched Laurie's tennis shoes, and off they went. Laurie ordered three scoops of different flavors of ice cream, with hot chocolate fudge, chopped nuts, and whipped cream. Bill had a vanilla cone. They ate the ice cream as they strolled back to their house.

Laurie's sweet tooth seemed insatiable that night. After she finished the ice cream, she ate several chocolates and sipped a snifter of cognac with them. Bill protested at the cognac. "That can't be good for the baby," he insisted, but Laurie dismissed the idea.

"That was earlier," she said. "The baby's all grown up now, and a little happy hour won't hurt."

They went to bed early, upstairs, and at Laurie's instigation, they made love for the first time since the night she'd gone into labor. Bill fretted at the idea, but not for too long; it had been nearly two months. Afterward, they snuggled, spoon fashion, and talked for a long time about nothing in particular.

Laurie woke before dawn and fairly leaped out of bed, humming and whistling as she padded naked around the bedroom and bathroom. She paused to examine herself in the full-length mirror; not exactly shapely, she decided, but not unattractive either. She looked closely and still couldn't see stretch marks. That was good; she'd still be able to wear a bikini.

After she dressed, she strolled down the hall to the room that would soon be the nursery and watched the beginnings of a sunrise through the lace curtains she'd insisted on putting in the room. Then she rearranged the furniture in the room, dusted, and tidied.

When Bill finally woke up, Laurie was downstairs, revamping the guest bedroom. She'd cleared out every sign that it had been her headquarters and their occasional bedroom for two months. She'd stripped the sheets and remade the king-size bed, and had carried all the legal documents upstairs, a box at a time, and stored them in the library. She was dusting everything when Bill came in, rubbing his eyes. "Are you crazy?" he asked.

"Probably," Laurie responded matter-of-factly. "I don't know why I feel so industrious. There must be *something* wrong with me. I should be dead tired."

Laurie had cooked and eaten a large breakfast, had finished cleaning the guest room, had tidied the rest of the downstairs, and was starting to vacuum the carpets when she felt the first contraction.

"Bill," she called. "Bill! Where are you?"

Bill stuck his head around a corner. "You touch my kitchen again," he said, "and I'll break your legs."

"Like hell you will," she said. "Bill, it's happening. I'm in labor. I just had a contraction."

"Omigod," Bill said, coming into the room. "Here we go again. Where's your bag?"

"Settle down," she said. "We've got a long time before we have to go to the hospital. I just wanted you to know."

"Not my fault," Bill said, holding up both hands. "Not my fault. That was—" he consulted his watch "—twelve-and-a-half hours ago."

"Dummy, that's not what I meant. It's okay this time. I'm thirty-nine weeks pregnant. It's *time* to have the baby. I'm gonna have a baby."

Hugging a woman who is nine months pregnant is an awkward exercise, but Bill managed it. He kissed Laurie, then drew his head back an inch and said softly, *"We're* going to have a baby. You can't take all the credit. I'm gonna help. Remember?" He let her go, took a step back, and looked her up and down appraisingly. "Okay," he said crisply. "Ready: Inhale! Exhale! Breathe! Breathe!" Then he dodged as Laurie lunged at him, claws extended.

"You'll get your chance, coach," she called after him. "But not yet." Bill disappeared around the corner, and Laurie, having nothing else to do, switched the vacuum cleaner back on and finished the living room rug. Then she sat down in her recliner.

Bill returned with two full champagne glasses, handed one to Laurie. She looked at the pale bubbly liquid wistfully, then started to hand it back. "I'd better not," she said.

"I know," Bill said, pulling a chair close to Laurie's. "It's ginger ale. Here's to the baby," he said holding his glass aloft. "Cheers."

They sipped ginger ale in silence for a few moments. Bill began to fidget, then said "Well? What do we do now?"

Laurie was at a loss. Everything they did, big or little, was always something goal-directed, a project to complete. The project now was having a baby, and for the next few hours it was going to be a part-time job. "We wait," she said finally. "Get the stopwatch and the chessboard."

The contractions, according to the stopwatch, occurred at intervals ranging at random between 15 minutes, 22 3/4 seconds and 12 minutes, 52 1/2 seconds. Laurie told Bill to put the stopwatch away.

They hadn't played chess in quite a while. Bill won the game in slightly less than an hour, despite playing around with the stopwatch. Laurie complained that he'd distracted her and that was why he'd won. Bill offered a rematch, but Laurie declined. She'd wait a few days, she said.

Laurie wasn't certain precisely when it would happen, but she knew her membranes ought to break sometime soon. She located her supply of sanitary napkins and put one in place. Then she and Bill went for a brief walk.

When they got back to the house, Bill brought out the stopwatch. The contractions ranged between eleven and thirteen minutes. Laurie groaned. "Last time, when we didn't want it to, it went faster," she complained.

When she later tried to describe the labor process, the thing she remembered most was the boredom. After the walk, she tried to relax for a while, but she was too restless to lounge in her recliner chair and she didn't want to lie on the bed for fear her membranes would break and soak everything. She and Bill played cards awhile, then switched to Trivial Pursuit, which Laurie won easily. When Bill offered to fix lunch, she declined. She wasn't hungry. By two o'clock in the afternoon, the contractions were seven minutes apart and growing stronger. They were uncomfortable, but not particularly painful. They went for another walk, but the contractions made Laurie's legs weak and she found herself grabbing Bill for support, or leaning against trees or fences until the contraction went away. It made her feel awkward, and it obviously made Bill nervous, so after they had walked once around the block, they went back into the house and played more card games.

When the contractions quickened to five-minute intervals, she phoned Dr. Crenshaw's answering service. Dr. Nagey returned the call. He sounded delighted to learn that Laurie was in labor. "Talk about great timing," he said. "You get to have your baby in the brand-new labor-and-delivery suite. We just moved up here this week. You're one of the few people to see both the old one and the new one. You'll appreciate the difference.

"Come on down whenever you're ready," he invited. "The place is deserted. It's a great afternoon to have a baby."

[22]

Labor . . .

TRISH, Laurie reflected on the way to the hospital, had been right. There was no experience quite like this. The contractions were coming regularly now, every five minutes, and yes, they were uncomfortable, even painful, but not unpleasantly so. It was the sort of wholesome ache that comes with the first long day of gardening every spring or the first few laps across the swimming pool in summer. It hurt, yes, but it did not feel at all unnatural. Laurie carefully noted each new contraction, compared it to the others, gauged the level of pain. Three, maybe four. No more.

What interested her more was the odd mixture of serenity and exhilaration she felt. She felt terribly alert, sensitive to tiny sounds and all the nuances of her body, but her heightened awareness was not accompanied by worry; she was calmly confident that everything was going precisely as it should.

Bill, on the other hand, was a nervous wreck. It was midafternoon on a Sunday, and the traffic was comparatively light, but Bill drove frantically, weaving and dodging, honking and swearing. Laurie double-checked her seat belt and repeatedly urged Bill to relax. They had plenty of time.

She'd been in labor about five hours now, by all calculations, and she still had some doubt whether this was the real thing. She'd read in her textbook about "false" labor, and she remembered that one of the ways to tell the real thing was whether the amniotic membranes have ruptured. Hers had not, and in the back of her mind she wondered if it was possible for true labor to begin before her water broke.

Besides, she'd expected to be in more pain than this. The contractions made her feel weak, but still, on her improvised scale of pain, it didn't hurt as much as she'd expected it to. She'd be embarrassed if she got to the hospital and Nagey sent her back home.

Heedless of all the "No Parking" signs, Bill pulled the car into the hospital's main driveway and stopped directly outside the entrance. He leaped out and ran around to open Laurie's door, and then, holding her duffel bag in one hand and her left arm in the other, he started for the glass doors.

"Wait," Laurie said sharply. She put an arm around Bill's back, leaned heavily against him, and took several deep breaths. "Okay," she said, relaxing. They walked briskly through the entranceway and toward the elevators. A uniformed guard looked up, nodded and smiled.

"I'll come move the car in a few minutes," Bill said as they walked past the guard.

"Take your time," the guard replied. "Business is real slow today."

There was even an elevator waiting for them, an experience unique among all Laurie's visits to University Hospital. Nagey was right, Laurie thought. It was going to be a very good day to have a baby.

Following Nagey's instructions, they went to the sixth floor. She and Bill walked, arm in arm, down the two long corridors toward the old delivery room. Nagey was waiting for them at the nurses' station in the octagonal rotunda of the old hospital building. He ushered them into one of the elevators that ringed the rotunda, and they silently rode up one floor.

The elevator doors opened, and the first thing Laurie noticed was the smell of fresh paint. She found herself in a small waiting area decorated in quiet beiges and bright primary colors, with soft chairs and a floor-to-ceiling mural of a woodland scene on one wall.

"Nice," she commented, looking around.

"This is just the beginning," Nagey said. "How far apart are your contractions?"

"Five minutes."

"Membranes break yet?"

"No."

"Good. We'll take the long way around." They walked a few steps down the hallway to a sliding door. A nurse at a glass-enclosed reception desk looked up, saw Nagey, and pushed a switch to open the doors.

Beyond those doors lay a beige corridor highlighted by bright orange and deep blue doors. It was as bright and fresh as the old delivery-suite hallway had been dark and gloomy.

The hallway was quiet, except for two women in the usual jade green scrub suits who stood outside one of the doorways, talking softly. They looked up, saw Nagey with Bill and Laurie, and walked toward them. "Aren't you Mrs. Edwards?" one of them asked.

"Yep," Laurie replied.

"I thought so," the nurse said. "I remember you. I was on duty when you were here before."

"This time it's not a drill," Laurie said.

"I know, but the routine's the same." The nurse held out her hand to Laurie, glancing at Nagey for confirmation.

"Give us two minutes," Nagey said to the nurse. "I'll bring her right back. I want to show off the new facilities a little."

The nurse winked at Laurie and Bill. "He helped design it," she said, nodding her head toward Nagey. "Now he wants to brag."

The tour took longer than two minutes. Nagey led them slowly along two wide, uncluttered hallways. Downstairs, the entire area had been littered with supply carts, shelves, boxes, and equipment. The new suites were spacious and efficient; even the omnipresent supply shelves had their own alcoves, and were encased in beige plastic cupboards with sliding covers.

The philosophy of the new delivery suite, Nagey explained, was to provide the least amount of medical intervention consistent with a safe delivery. He led Laurie and Bill along a row of private birthing rooms, the rooms where normal, uncomplicated labor and delivery would take place. "That's a change," Nagey said. "Downstairs, you had your labor in one place, and then moved to the delivery room to have the baby. Here we won't do that unless there's a reason."

Each room contained a single birthing bed, a specially designed hospital bed. Nagey led them into an empty room to demonstrate one of the beds. It resembled a normal hospital bed, but it had a colonial-style oak headboard, and the side rails were also made of wood.

"No stirrups?" Laurie asked.

"Don't usually need them," Nagey answered. "We do keep them around," he said, "but not too many mothers ask for them."

They walked back down the hall, with Nagey pointing out various specialized areas. There were old-style delivery rooms for the difficult cases, and operating rooms for cesarean sections and the like. There were consultation rooms and supply rooms, anesthesia rooms, and even a small conference room equipped with a tiny kitchen.

Then they returned to the nurses' station, where Laurie's nurse was waiting. "Last stop," Nagey said, "is the admitting room. This one's newer and nicer than the one downstairs, but that's all that's different."

"Come on, hon," the nurse said, leading Laurie toward the examining room, "we'll get you through all the preliminaries and let you change into one of our world-famous designer gowns."

When Bill went off to park the car, the nurse collected a urine specimen and blood sample from Laurie, took her temperature and blood pressure, and gave her a second open-at-the-back hospital gown to go over the first. "Put this one on backward," she counseled. "You don't feel so undressed that way."

Shortly, Dr. Nagey walked into the examining room. "What do you think?" he asked brightly.

"You're right, some things never change," she agreed. "I guess now we just wait. My membranes still haven't ruptured yet," she reported, using the physicians' phrasing. "I guess that means we'll be a while."

"Not necessarily," Nagey said. "Some babies are born with membranes still intact. It's an old good-luck charm to be 'born wearing a caul'—it was supposed to be an infallible protection from drowning. Nowadays we usually break the membranes ourselves to put in a monitor or just to speed things up a little."

As he talked, he began pressing his hands against Laurie's abdomen, checking the baby's position. He had been routinely checking the baby's position for several months. Until now, the position had been all but irrelevant; now that Laurie was in labor, it was vitally important.

A baby's body is designed to pass through the birth canal headfirst, with its chin on its chest and the back of its head emerging first. That normal "vertex" presentation occurs in better than ninety-five percent of all deliveries. If Laurie's baby was a breech or shoulder presentation, or, worst of all, a transverse lie, with the back across the birth canal, Nagey wanted to know it now. If the baby was in a dangerous position, they would do a cesarean section.

Like the pelvic exam, this was an old, familiar routine for Nagey. Anything out of the ordinary would focus his attention instantly, and if he suddenly got very quiet, Laurie would start to worry. But Nagey continued talking casually about the amniotic membranes. "One department chairman out in St. Louis," he said, "posted a notice to all residents that he would pay fifty dollars to any resident who delivered a baby inside intact membranes. Well, he got four of them the first week, and he had to withdraw the offer before he went broke."

Standing beside the examining table, Nagey pressed his hands against the sides of Laurie's abdomen. He could feel vague, irregular lumps on her left side, and a long, flat surface on her right. That was perfect. The lumps were most likely the baby's legs and bottom, and the flat surface the baby's back. That would mean the baby was in the right position.

"We've never made an offer like that here," he went on. "Nobody wanted to put up the fifty dollars. But we like to tell that story to the residents to make the point that if you don't *have* to do it, you probably shouldn't do it. Most of the time, the best thing you can do is keep your cotton-pickin' hands off.''

With his right hand, he squeezed Laurie's abdomen just above her pubis. He could feel the hard roundness of the baby's head. More reassurance. Better still, the head did not move as he pressed against it. That meant Laurie was in active labor, that the baby's head was already working its way through the cervical canal.

"In just a minute, I'll check your cervix and see how far it's dilated,'' he said. "Then we'll have a good idea of how much longer you've got to go. How are the contractions? Are you having any great discomfort?''

"Nowhere near what I expected,'' Laurie said. "It hurts, but not that badly.''

"Good.'' Nagey turned and, facing Laurie's feet, pressed his hands against both sides of the lower part of her abdomen, feeling for the baby's forehead. It was where it belonged, on the side opposite the baby's back. The baby's chin was against its chest, as it should be.

The tests he had performed, known as Leopold's maneuvers, are more than a century old, but Nagey preferred them to the impersonal technology of the ultrasound machine. There was an ultrasound machine handy, and if any of the tests had raised any doubts in his mind, he would have immediately confirmed his suspicions with a quick scan; but whenever possible he liked to keep the technology in the background, available if needed, but otherwise ignored.

"I need to check your cervix,'' he said, with a note of apology in his voice, "but I want to wait and do it when you have your next contraction. I can tell a lot more during a contraction than I can otherwise. Unfortunately, it's also about the most uncomfortable time for you that I could possibly do it.''

"I don't mind,'' Laurie said, then caught herself. "Actually I'll probably mind it a lot, but do it anyway. I understand.'' They chatted a few moments longer, until Laurie felt another contraction beginning. "Okay, go ahead,'' she told Nagey.

He was right, the exam was uncomfortable, very uncomfortable. With Nagey's fingers pushing against her from one side and the baby's head pushing from the other side, the pain shot up to a six, at least, but when Nagey withdrew his fingers, it went back down to the same three or four it had been all along. Laurie took several deep breaths.

"You're not going to believe this," Nagey said. "But you're already about seven centimeters dilated. How long have you been in labor?"

"About five hours," Laurie said.

"That's remarkable for a first pregnancy," Nagey said. "You're going to have this baby sooner than I would have guessed. Most first labors last twelve or fourteen hours, minimum. You're probably going to get out with less than that."

"It's probably that dress rehearsal I had a few weeks ago," Laurie observed.

Nagey looked thoughtful. "You're probably right. I'm sure that makes a difference." He took out Laurie's charts and began writing. In terse medical jargon he recorded the observations he had just made, and added a note for future reference: Laurie's labor had been rapid and relatively painless, and had been preceded by an episode of premature labor. None of that was particularly abnormal, but it was enough to make Nagey wonder, in passing, if Laurie's cervix might be just a little less firm than it ought to be. The worry was most likely unfounded, he knew, but just in case, he wrote that in future pregnancies it might be a good idea to check Laurie's cervix regularly.

He did not mention his suspicion to Laurie; there was no need. She was at term, in normal labor, with no apparent complications. He'd bring it up two days from now, when she would be ready to go home. No point worrying her now, when things were going so well.

"Some people have all the luck," he commented instead to Laurie. "Not only are you going to have a short labor and, from what I can tell, a very nice delivery, you also get to use the VIP birthing room."

"The VIP birthing room?"

"C'mon," he said, beckoning her down off the examining table. "I'll show you."

Nagey walked out into the hall and spoke briefly to Bill, who had returned from the garage. When Laurie joined them, he led the two of them down the long corridor past the row of birthing rooms they'd seen before. At the far end, he pushed open a door, and Laurie stared, amazed. The room was lit by the soft glow of a table lamp. She could see an armchair, and a rocking chair, beside another oak-trimmed birthing bed that had been adjusted and tilted so that it looked more like a chaise lounge than a bed. On the wall opposite the bed, a small herd of deer grazed contentedly in another floor-to-ceiling woodland mural. "Through the wonders of modern medical engineering," Nagey said, grinning, "you get to have your baby the old-fashioned way."

"I'm gonna recommend you to all my friends," Laurie said, climbing gingerly onto the bed. "This looks like fun. Where's the gearshift?"

Nagey showed her the controls. "Find a position that's comfortable for you," he instructed. "I want to put a monitor on you for a little while, and you'll need to be as still as possible then."

Nagey disappeared, and shortly afterward a nurse and a resident came in. They strapped a pair of large sensors across her abdomen to monitor the fetus. The resident flipped a switch and the machine, which hung from the ceiling in a corner of the room, began tracing black zigzags along the moving strip of paper.

"We want to leave it on for ten or fifteen minutes," the resident told her, "so we can get several contractions. This thing is very sensitive to your movements, so try not to move any more than you absolutely have to." Laurie nodded her head, and the needles jumped. "That's what I mean," the resident said.

Laurie lay as still as she could, but she found that it was almost impossible to avoid moving during a contraction. Bill sat in the rocking chair with his stopwatch and fidgeted between contractions. They were four minutes apart now. The nurse and the resident watched awhile, then quietly left.

After awhile, Nagey returned. "Everything okay?" he asked. Laurie started to answer, then stiffened as another contraction began. Nagey leaned over the bed and gently tested her abdomen with one hand. "You're looking good," he commented, and turned to examine the strip of paper protruding from the monitor. Starting at the far end, he let his eye run along the zigzag line tracing the fetal heart rate, looking for late decelerations. There were none . . . or were there? There was a lot of "noise" after the two most recent contractions, but when the line had settled back into its normal zigzag pattern, it seemed slightly lower, and then it had moved up slightly. Laurie had just finished another contraction and now, while Nagey watched, the pattern was repeated.

He straightened, turned back to Laurie and Bill. "The television works, if you're in the mood," he said, nodding at the TV that hung in one corner of the room. "It's too late for baseball, but 'Sixty Minutes' will be on in a little while."

"Good," Bill said.

"Am I going to have time to watch it?" Laurie asked.

"Probably," Nagey answered. "Want me to check?"

"Sure."

Nagey walked to the foot of the bed, pulled on an examining glove, and gingerly inspected Laurie's cervix, avoiding the amniotic membrane that now bulged through the opening. "Still a little way to go," he said. "If I break the membrane it might speed things up."

"Then please do," Laurie said. On her scale of one to ten, the pain had gone up from four to five, and now it was, she judged, about a six. Bearable, but not something she wanted to endure any longer than necessary.

"Hold very still now." With a long, pointed instrument, Nagey carefully pierced the membrane. Suddenly, Laurie felt a gush of warm liquid. She fought the impulse to move. "Now I've made a mess," she complained.

Nagey stood up, grinned at her. "Goes with the territory," he said. "Hard to have a baby without it." He pulled off the plastic gloves and dropped them in a trashcan. "Lie as still as you can for the next couple of contractions. I want to get a little more tracing on the monitor."

Bill moved the rocking chair alongside the bed and held Laurie's hand while they watched the local news. Nagey came in quietly and studied the lengthening strip of paper coming out of the monitor. Finally, he cleared his throat. "I'm a tiny bit concerned about these readings," he said. "It could be just the monitor, but there seem to be some drops in the baby's heart rate that we don't like to see. There's no cause for alarm, but if you don't mind, I'd like to switch to an internal monitor probe. It gives much more reliable readings."

"Whatever you think," Laurie said. Bill nodded agreement.

Nagey disappeared briefly, returned carrying a plastic tube with a twist of red and green wires coming out of one end. "This," he said, "is the internal monitor. This has a clip that attaches directly to the baby's scalp. This will eliminate a lot of the noise we've been getting on the monitor."

He moved back to the foot of the bed and, pulling on a new pair of gloves, threaded the tube up inside Laurie until he felt it touch the top of the baby's head. He twisted a knob on the tube with his left hand, and at the far end, a tiny steel clip pierced the outer layer of the baby's scalp, securing the monitor in place. Nagey withdrew the applicator tube and taped the wires to Laurie's leg. Then he disconnected the cable from the device on Laurie's abdomen and connected it to the internal monitor. The needle, which had swung wildly during the procedure, settled back into its customary zigzag line.

"I need you to do one more thing for me," Nagey said. As the nurse unstrapped the external monitors from Laurie's abdomen, Nagey took out a clear plastic oxygen mask and connected it to a fixture on the wall. "Before I do any worrying, I want to satisfy myself that you're getting plenty of oxygen. What I want you to do is lie on your right side and breathe through the mask for a few minutes, okay?'' He handed the mask to Laurie. "I'll be back.''

Laurie rolled onto her side and put the mask in place. She could still see the television, but the mask muffled her voice, so she and Bill watched television in silence, with the monitor humming in the background. They had attempted conversation several times, but nothing they could think to talk about seemed terribly important. The umpteenth time Bill had asked "How do you feel?'' Laurie had snapped "Lousy!'' She had apologized immediately, but Bill had stopped asking. Laurie had wanted something to drink—she still wasn't hungry—and the nurse had returned with a cup of ice chips. Laurie chewed on the ice, handing the cup to Bill each time she had a contraction. The pain was a little worse, a six, maybe a seven now. She'd found that crossing her arms and hugging herself seemed to help, and so did breathing deeply. The contractions were only about three minutes apart now, and one particularly strong spasm made Laurie groan with pain. Bill said nothing, but reached a hand up and lightly caressed her abdomen, moving his fingertips around and around in widening circles. Almost instantly, Laurie relaxed, and let out a long breath. "Oooh, that's nice,'' she said softly. The television program continued, unwatched, as Bill swiveled his chair so he could continue stroking Laurie with one hand while he held the stopwatch in the other.

Nagey returned and studied the monitor tracing. The tracing was much cleaner now, and it clearly showed shallow dips in the fetal heart rate after contractions. "This is not terribly alarming,'' he told Bill and Laurie, pointing to the tracing, "but it's enough to make me cautious. What I would like to do is take a tiny blood sample from the baby's scalp. That will tell us very reliably whether the baby's in any trouble. Unfortunately, it's also a somewhat uncomfortable test.''

"I'm uncomfortable already,'' Laurie said. "I don't suppose a little more will do any harm.''

"Jeez, what a nice patient you are,'' Nagey said admiringly. "You haven't yelled at me once yet.''

"No," she said, forcing a smile, "I yell at Bill instead." Bill grinned and squeezed her hand.

"Tonight, you can yell at anybody you want to." Nagey said with a grin. "I'll be right back." Less than a minute later, he was back, accompanied by a nurse and two residents. "You won't enjoy this," he predicted, "so I'll be as quick as I can."

While the nurse swabbed brown antiseptic between Laurie's legs, Nagey pulled on a pair of sterile gloves and then nodded to one of the residents, who broke open a small package and held it out to him. Nagey reached a gloved hand into the package and took out a white plastic cone. He held it out so Laurie could see it.

"This is the undignified part," he said. "I'm going to have one of the residents hold your left leg up in the air so I can put in this little cone to get access to the baby's scalp. Ready?"

Laurie grunted assent through the oxygen mask, and one of the residents hoisted her leg into the air. Nagey sat on a stool beside the bed, and the other resident stood beside him waiting for orders.

With his left hand, Nagey parted Laurie's labia and slid the cone inward, gently applying increasing pressure until the tip of the cone touched the baby's scalp, right beside the monitor probe. Laurie panted through clenched teeth, but said nothing.

At a word from Nagey, the resident beside him lifted a small plastic bottle, maneuvered it into place, and squirted a few drops of volatile liquid onto the baby's scalp. As the liquid evaporated it chilled the skin, and blood rushed to the surface. Nagey held out his hand and the resident handed him a tiny, long-handled scalpel.

Nagey eased the scalpel into the plastic cone and carefully made a tiny nick in the scalp. A drop of blood welled up immediately. Nagey exchanged the scalpel for a long glass pipette and drew out an almost microscopic sample of the baby's blood. He handed the pipette to the resident and withdrew the plastic cone. Laurie took several deep breaths, but she still said nothing.

"All done," Nagey said. The resident left, carrying the pipette. "Results momentarily. You can take off the mask now, by the way."

Laurie was still breathing heavily. "You were right," she finally said. "That was . . . uncomfortable. I'm ready to get this over with."

"Soon," Nagey promised. "Soon."

In a small laboratory just down the hall, the resident put the pipette into an electronic pH meter. The machine had already been turned on, calibrated, and set up for this test, but the resident glanced at the lighted "ready" indicator to be sure. Testing the acidity of the baby's blood was the surest way to tell if the baby was getting enough oxygen. If the baby was deprived of oxygen, its cells would begin to dump lactic acid into the bloodstream, lowering the blood pH from its normal 7.3 to 7.4 range. If Laurie's baby proved to have a blood pH of 7.2 or lower, the resident would call the standby anesthesiologist even before he returned to the birthing room.

As soon as the sample was in place, the machine performed the pH test automatically, and the resident glanced at the electronic readout as he tore off the strip of paper that the machine had also printed out. The printout always said exactly the same thing as the readout, but the resident always checked. They matched. With the strip of paper in his hand, the resident turned and walked out into the hallway.

He walked back to the birthing room, where Nagey still chatted with Laurie and Bill. The resident stood in the doorway until Nagey noticed him. "Seven-three-three," he said simply.

"That means everything's fine," Nagey said to Laurie and Bill. "I'm going to leave the monitor on, just in case, but it looks like everything's going fine." Nagey saw Laurie's face contort as another contraction started. "Deep breaths," he reminded Laurie. "Deep breaths. Don't forget how to relax," he said. Bill resumed caressing Laurie's abdomen. The contraction passed.

"I think I would've almost been grateful for a C-section," Laurie muttered.

Nagey chuckled. "You missed your chance. However, if it gets too bad, there's always an epidural. If you're going to want one, now's the time to make up your mind. Once you go into transition, it's too late.''

Laurie thought a moment. It was a real temptation. The pain had become much more intense in the last hour, easily a six or a seven, and at that she might have set her imaginary scale too low. And she felt tired, weak, almost ill. Still—she remembered Trish's warning that anesthetics blunted the exhiliration as well as the pain.

''No,'' she said finally, ''I don't want to miss all the fun.''

[23]

. . . And Delivery

LAURIE hurt constantly now, and the pain ranged from an aching, burning soreness between contractions to excruciating cramps whenever another one started. Some contractions were worse than others; sometimes the pain shot up to what she thought must be the limit, ten on a scale of ten, and in her mind she began to panic. It was too soon, she thought, too soon for such pain. Something must be wrong; she felt strained to the limit and beyond, felt like her insides must surely explode in the next instant.

The contractions came rapidly, almost continuously, and Laurie found herself struggling for breath. Bill stood rigidly beside the bed, quietly stroking Laurie's abdomen, her hips, her shoulders, murmuring things Laurie couldn't quite understand. When the contractions came, he would whisper "Deep breaths! Deep breaths!" with a note of urgency in his voice. Laurie found herself becoming annoyed. Deep breaths hurt, she complained to herself. Why the hell couldn't he see that? Several times she pushed him away from her, but he always came back.

Most of her consciousness now belonged to a great numbing presence, powerful but inarticulate, and Laurie knew that it, not she, was in control. Her mind refused to focus; Bill's voice, and even his touch, seemed distant. Reality consisted only of herself and the pain.

Slowly at first, and then with increasing urgency, Laurie realized with horror that her bowel had suddenly become full, full to bursting, and she needed desperately to defecate. Oh, why hadn't they given her an enema before? Why did they let this happen?

She felt her sphincter muscle begin to dilate. Fighting to keep it intact, she struggled to sit up. *No!* she thought fiercely. She would *not* soil the bed; she would *not* be humiliated, she would *not* lose control! She would have her bowel movement in the bathroom! Bill's hands pushed against her shoulders, gently at first, then harder, harder, until she lost her balance and fell back against the bed. "No, no," he was saying, "you stay right there."

"Bill, you don't understand," she whispered desperately, "I've got to get up."

"You can't get up," answered Bill's voice, "you stay right where you are."

The frustration mounted higher and higher. "Goddammit, Bill, I've got to shit!" she wailed. Why couldn't he understand? What the hell kind of husband was he, anyway?

"No you don't," the voice answered, "that's the baby. The baby's coming down now. Don't fight it; bear down." Bill still had one hand on Laurie's shoulder, but now the voice was Nagey's.

Laurie felt surrounded, captive. Deep in her mind, the old horror fantasies stirred. She felt helpless, and helplessness meant failure. She fought for control. "I have been defecating all my life," she announced as crisply as she could, "and I know what it feels like. Either you let me up, or I will defecate on this bed."

She heard the voice chuckle. "Don't worry about it; we're ready for it if you do. Everybody does it. You can't have a baby without it."

The anger peaked, then subsided as the tiny speck of reason in her mind whispered, "Go ahead. Do what they say. Bear down hard. Blow it all the way across the room, if you can. Then let them laugh." At the next contraction, she set her teeth and put every ounce of effort she could muster into tightening her abdomen. She felt her sphincter open, but the pain began to mount, and grow worse, and worse, until she could feel no sensation but the pain. Finally it became unbearable and she relaxed, panting. The pain receded, almost went away.

"Wonderful," Nagey's voice said. "That was absolutely wonderful. Do that again, and you'll have a baby." The words swept away Laurie's mental fog. She looked up and saw Bill's face. She closed her eyes again as he wiped her face with a cool washcloth. She brushed a hand across her forehead and realized her hair was damp with sweat.

"Look at me," she complained softly. "I'm a mess."

"You're gorgeous," Bill said unsteadily.

"You're crazy," she said, smiling.

"You're both doing just fine," Nagey added from the end of the bed.

Laurie lifted her head slightly and appraised the situation. The birthing bed was tilted so that, even though she was lying on her back, her head was substantially higher than her feet. Instead of being strapped into stirrups, her feet were set against the edge of the footrest, while her bottom hung slightly over the precipice where the footrest was detached from the bed, exposing a hollow, plastic-lined space below. Her knees were wide apart, she noted absently, thinking about a time not long ago when she'd have been scandalized to assume such a position in front of witnesses. Now it didn't seem at all out of the ordinary.

Another contraction started. The pain ran quickly back up the scale from severe to excruciating to unbearable. Laurie strained with all her might, while Nagey stood at the end of the bed calling "That's it. Push. Push. Push," and Bill leaned close to her and whispered, "C'mon, you can do it, you can do it. Push."

The pain peaked and held, and Laurie let out a strangled groan through her clenched teeth. "Pant!" Nagey shouted. "Shallow breaths! Pant like a puppy dog." Laurie gasped, panted. Miraculously, the pain lessened slightly. "Push!" Nagey said. "Push some more. Push more. Push."

The pain reached unbearable again, hung there a moment, then receded as the contraction stopped. Laurie lay bathed in sweat, gasping for breath. Her body trembled with the recollection of the pain.

"The baby almost came out that time," Nagey reported. "Next time ought to be it. Save up every ounce of strength you've got and give me the biggest push you can."

Laurie lay still, breathing heavily. The pain had shifted now from her abdomen to her perineum, the region between her legs;

it was a sharp soreness, coupled with an overwhelming feeling of fullness and pressure—almost, she thought, like the most terrible constipation you could imagine. She immediately felt guilty, and chastised herself for the thought. This was her *baby* goddammit. Bill wiped her face with the damp cloth again, and she looked up at him and smiled. "You okay?" she asked.

"No," Bill answered with his poker face.

"Good," Laurie replied. "Why should I do all the suffering? You take the next contraction, okay?"

Bill grinned. "Gee, I'd love to, but . . . " he let the sentence trail off.

"You'll get yours. Wait and see. Uh-oh, here it comes." Laurie felt the contraction begin, and she could tell it was a big one. She opened her mouth and began panting, forcing herself to relax. She'd formulated her strategy for this one even while she chatted with Bill, and the first requirement was to relax. The pain worsened, worsened, and she breathed in small, shallow gasps, concentrating with all her will, forcing herself to stay relaxed, stay relaxed until the contraction hit its peak. This was the big one; it grew, and it grew, until the pain was a stabbing, burning, breathtaking ten. The pain filled all her consciousness, but still her mind was clear. *This was it.*

"Hold on to me," she told Bill. She took an enormous breath, set her teeth, and began to bear down. The pain, as bad as the worst she could ever have imagined, grew worse, an eleven, a twelve. A growl escaped through her teeth, became a groan, but still she pushed, and the pain got worse, thirteen, fourteen. The groan became a yell, a wail, a primal, inarticulate scream as the pain exploded like lightening inside her brain, off the scale, unmeasurable, and then, magically, in one long, shuddering breath, dropped to zero.

It was done. Laurie relaxed, shivered, and almost fainted. She became aware that Bill was hugging her, his face against hers, kissing her cheek.

"Gorgeous. Wonderful. Best I've seen in a long time," Laurie heard Nagey say, from the end of the bed. "Now do me a favor, Laurie. Whatever you do, *don't push any more for a min-*

226 / Autumn's Children

ute. Give me a minute to get organized down here.'' The words were calm, jovial, friendly. Laurie heard nothing amiss in his voice as he added, apparently not to her, ''Hemostats.''

Nagey quietly thanked fate that Laurie didn't ask for the mirror. No need to frighten anyone else. If the mirror had been set up, Laurie would be looking as Nagey was, at the baby's head, facing the floor, eyes tightly closed, slowly turning purple as the umbilical cord around its neck strangled it.

As the head had come out, Nagey had slipped his left hand under it to support it. He'd been in the middle of complimenting Laurie when the neck emerged and he saw the cord. In the same instant that he spoke the word ''hemostats,'' he slipped a gloved finger under the cord and reached out his right hand. A nurse instantly laid the clamp in it, and he snapped it onto the cord. He held out his hand again, applied the second clamp to the cord. ''Scissors,'' he said. The practiced tone of voice was as calm as if he'd been discussing the afternoon's baseball game. Only the nurse could see the tension in his face.

With the clamps in place, he lifted the cord a fraction farther from the baby's neck, maneuvered the scissors under it, and snipped. The cord, weighted by the stainless-steel clamps on either side of Nagey's finger, fell away from the baby's neck. The clamps clattered together somewhere below the baby's face. The procedure had taken five, perhaps ten seconds.

Nagey visibly relaxed. ''Okay,'' he said to the nurse, ''*Now* the syringe.'' The syringe was a rubber bulb like a miniature baster, and with his left hand, Nagey gently moved the baby's head around until it was facing Laurie's right thigh. Moving rapidly but deliberately, he squeezed the bulb, put the tip into one of the baby's nostrils, and released the bulb. He repeated the operation for the other nostril, and then a third time for the baby's mouth. As soon as Nagey removed the rubber syringe, the baby coughed twice, then began to cry softly. Nagey felt the surge of elation welling up in his chest, and he took a long, slow breath to steady himself. ''Hear that?'' he asked Laurie. ''That's your baby.''

At the other end of the bed, Bill had bathed Laurie's face again, and with one hand Laurie worked uselessly at arranging her hair. The pain had vanished, had been replaced by a euphoria and heightened awareness unlike anything Laurie had ever felt before. She could hear the baby's cries, of course, but it wasn't really crying, she knew. There was no fright in it; it sounded more like singing than crying. She could hear tiny sounds from the other end of the hallway, could discriminate among the myriad smells of a hospital and identify the individual ones. From somewhere, amid all the antiseptic odors, came the aroma of fried chicken.

"Boy, am I hungry," Laurie observed. "When do we eat?"

She heard Nagey chuckle. "First things first," he said. "Let's finish having this baby. You can give me a little push now." The baby's shoulders had rotated until they were vertical, for the easiest exit. Laurie felt a contraction, squeezed a bit, and the baby squirted out into Nagey's waiting hands.

"Nine-oh-one," a nurse said aloud.

"Nine-oh-one," another nurse repeated, and left the room to log the delivery.

Nagey held the baby up like a trophy. "You," he said with great ceremony, "have a daughter."

Epilogue

Fortieth birthdays are not always joyful occasions, but Laurie's was. It was a combination birthday celebration, family reunion, and belated baby shower. Laurie's parents, Bill's parents, as many grandparents as could travel, and a crowd of aunts, uncles, cousins, nephews, and nieces gathered in Baltimore for a feast that began before noon one Sunday and went on until well after dark. One of the guests of honor, Kimberly Elaine Edwards, aged seven months, slept contentedly through most of the festivities.

Almost as soon as Laurie got home from the hospital, she resumed working a part-time schedule at her law firm, and will continue that way until Kimberly is no longer nursing. Laurie offered to take an unpaid leave from the firm, but her partners would not hear of it; her knowledge of business law, they said, was too valuable to lose. So she works mornings at the office and then brings her paperwork home. Sometimes she sits in the sunlit nursery, rocking gently, reading the latest antitrust cases while she breastfeeds her daughter.

After the baby was born, Laurie got a new diaphragm and began using it, but lately she and Bill have begun to talk about having a second child. After all, they say, forty isn't as old as it used to be.

Author's Postscript

Shortly after the manuscript for this book was completed, Dr. Crenshaw stopped smoking.

Bibliography

Nagey, D. A.; Pupkin, M. J.; MacKenna, J.; Schomberg, D. W.; and Crenshaw, M. C., Jr. "A physiologic model of the dehydroepiandrosterone to estrogen conversion system in the fetoplacental unit. I. Development." *American Journal of Obstetrics and Gynecology* 125(2):249-55 (5/15/76).

Nagey, D. A.; Pupkin, M. J.; Mandeville, L.; Schomberg, D. W.; and Crenshaw, M. C., Jr. "The dehydroepiandrosterone loading test. IV. Evaluation of clinical utility." *American Journal of Obstetrics and Gynecology* 142(1):60-65 (1/1/82).

Netter, F. H. *Reproductive System.* Vol. 2 of *The Ciba Collection of Medical Illustrations.* Summit, NJ: Ciba Pharmaceutical Co., 1965.

Niswander, Kenneth R. *Obstetrics: Essentials of Clinical Practice,* 2d ed. Boston: Little, Brown, 1981.

Pritchard, J. A., and MacDonald, P. C. *Williams Obstetrics,* 16th ed. New York: Appleton-Century-Crofts, 1976.

Pupkin, M. J.; Nagey, D. A.; MacKenna, J.; Schomberg, D. W.; and Crenshaw, M. C., Jr. "A physiologic model of the dehydroepiandrosterone to estrogen conversion system in the fetoplacental unit. II. Preliminary clinical application—the dehydroepiandrosterone loading test." *American Journal of Obstetrics and Gynecology* 125(2):256-62 (5/15/76).

Pupkin, M. J.; Nagey, D. A.; Schomberg, D. W.; MacKenna, J.; and Crenshaw, M. C., Jr. "The dehydroepiandrosterone loading test. III. A possible placental function test." *American Journal of Obstetrics and Gynecology* 134(3):281-88 (6/1/79).

Rovinsky, J. J. "Management of Normal Labor and Delivery." Chap. 65 in *Clinical Obstetrics.* Vol. 2 of *Obstetrics and Gynecology,* revised ed. Philadelphia: Harper & Row, 1984.

Silbar, E. L., "Psychoprophylactic Preparation for Childbirth." Chap. 20 in *Clinical Obstetrics.* Vol. 2 of *Obstetrics and Gynecology,* revised ed. Philadelphia: Harper & Row, 1984.

Sokol, R. J., and D'Angelo, L. "Fetal Monitoring During Labor." Chap. 58 in *Clinical Obstetrics.* Vol. 2 of *Obstetrics and Gynecology,* revised ed. Philadelphia: Harper & Row, 1984.